Wack
Addicted to Internet Porn

WACK

Addicted to Internet Porn
By Noah B.E. Church

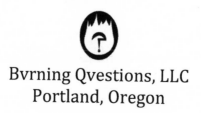

Bvrning Qvestions, LLC
Portland, Oregon

Contents

Introduction

I am no right-wing fundamentalist, preacher, or born-again porn star. What I am is a man who regularly used Internet porn from age 9 until age 24—most of my life. In all that time I had no moral objection to pornography. I believed I was living in a time in which people were free to explore their innate sexuality, and porn was one natural and healthy outlet of that freedom. I was wrong about that part.

It was only several months ago that I fully understood the damage pornography had done to my sexual and emotional health. I was a porn addict, even at only a few uses each week. I did not realize until then that porn was not just another pastime: habitual porn use over years had physiologically altered me, rewiring my brain to respond only to increasingly extreme and constantly changing porn clips, rendering me physically unable to maintain an erection with a real woman or have any semblance of enjoyable sex. Exposure to an unlimited amount of beautiful women on my computer fooled my sexual response system into thinking that I was getting an endless supply of attractive mates willing to do anything I wanted. This does not happen in nature (sorry, guys). Thus my brain was treated to unnaturally frequent and powerful releases of several neurochemicals—most notably dopamine, which is a neurotransmitter responsible for immediate craving, desire, and motivation to pursue something evolutionarily advantageous to our survival (fatty foods, good sex). This dopamine overload desensitized me to real-life stimulation, emotionally and sexually deadening me and destroying my sexual confidence as well as every romantic relationship I ever had.

It did not take much research to discover that many, many men—and many women, too—were having similar problems, some less extreme and some more so. But there were also people who viewed porn happily without noticing any related issues. Like alcohol it seemed that some people can use recreationally and still maintain a normal, healthy lifestyle while others—especially those who masturbate to deal with stress or difficult emotions—can come to use porn habitually. If not interrupted, the habit becomes an addiction that can cause sexual, emotional, and social dysfunction. And like all addictions porn can be extremely difficult to leave behind, as the following man testifies.

Anonymous: *I've battled a few addictions in my life—from nicotine to alcohol and other substances. I've overcome all of them, and this was by far the most* *difficult. Urges, crazy thoughts, sleeplessness, feelings of hopelessness, despair, worthlessness, and many more negative things were all part of what I went through. [...] This recovery required a will beyond what I thought I was capable of...and I do have a pretty strong will—I do give myself credit for that. I always manage to right the ship and stay the course, and I have crawled out of some pretty dark places in my life. But, again...with this, I really thought all hope was lost. Really. Really. Really.*

A growing number of people like this man were telling their stories of porn addiction and recovery on the Internet, forming communities of mutual support and challenging one another to break the addictive cycle. They called this endeavor "no PMO" (for Porn, Masturbation, Orgasm) or "NoFap" (fapping is slang for masturbation). Those who were successful enjoyed a complete reversal of the problems that brought them to those communities, and many of them experienced a myriad of improvements in areas of their lives that they had no idea had been damaged by their porn habits. For the most part these were not people who were morally against sexual expression or masturbation. In fact they very much wanted to live enjoyable sex lives, but they had found that porn use and chronic masturbation were holding them back.

As I read these accounts and more formal research studies on porn's influence over us, it became clear to me that porn changes people in many ways both subtle and overt—and not for the better. If you are like I was a year ago, then that statement will offend you. In fact, many moments in this book can be very uncomfortable and disturbing to confront, especially if you use porn and can see how this information applies to your life. I write bluntly about subjects few people ever have the courage or inclination to talk about, and it can be shocking. But do not be disheartened. I do not share these facts to show that the porn addict's situation is hopeless—quite the opposite. I share these facts to demonstrate just how much we can improve our lives by leaving addiction behind. So when you read something in this book that strikes too close to home, making you want to turn away and forget in the spirit of blissful ignorance, remember that the problems discussed in this text are for the most part entirely reversible, and former compulsive porn users often report enjoying happiness, self-respect, and quality relationships at a level they never knew was possible.

When I say "porn" or "pornography" I am referring to any material—written, pictorial, cinematic, digital, phone/chat sex, etc.—

that is produced for the purpose of eliciting sexual excitement. Addiction to porn is not new, but never before the Internet age has it been so easy and cheap for most of the developed world to acquire any type and degree of pornographic material, and this change has especially impacted our youth, who are often more computer-literate and able to access hardcore porn than their parents.

The first part of this book explores the data currently available about how Internet porn affects its consistent users. This may be valuable to you whether you use porn yourself or know someone who does (and unless you live in an extremely isolated, Internet-free community, you know people who use porn). In order to provide more personal perspectives on these facts, I frequently include in italics the words of men and women who have decided to share their stories.

Much of the following scientific information was originally featured on "www.yourbrainonporn.com", an excellent source of education on aspects of porn addiction. This website is created and maintained by Gary Wilson and Marnia Robinson. Wilson is a retired professor of anatomy, physiology, and pathology, and his "passion is the neuroscience of reward, sex, and bonding." In addition to the many articles and videos the pair has made on porn addiction, Wilson gave a presentation called "The Great Porn Experiment", which with more than two million views on YouTube has helped bring this subject into the public dialogue.

The second part of this book is directed specifically toward men who realize that porn use has done significant enough damage to their lives that they want to make a change—but are not sure how. Men make up the bulk of porn addicts and so I write to them, but there are many women who also struggle with this problem and want to change. While there are neurological differences between men and women that affect how we interact with porn, at the same time we all function on the same basic emotional principles, and most information and recovery tactics I give apply equally as well to women.

I said that I am no preacher, and neither am I a psychologist, neuroscientist, or sex counselor. My words should not be considered the opinion of any profession. What I am is a man inspired by his own struggles to scour the Earth for reliable information and anecdotes about porn addiction and recovery. When I give facts, I link to their appropriate references, but the truth is that the scientific and medical community has yet to catch up to a problem that has reached epidemic proportions and has the capacity to ruin lives, and I feel the need to help others combat this problem now rather than to wait for more long-term, peer-reviewed studies to be conducted. Therefore much of the information concerning recovery is collected from anecdotes, informal experiments, and personal experience. Read it as such.

Part One: The Problem

Wired to be an addict
(neuropathology of porn addiction)

In order to understand how a behavior like viewing porn can cause physical changes to our brains and lead to addiction, the first fact that needs to be recognized is that the brain is plastic (neuroplasticity). This does not mean that the brain can be recycled alongside our juice cartons and newspapers. Rather, neuroplasticity refers to the fact that our brains can grow and change throughout our lives. The brain may change for a variety of reasons, such as accommodating substance additions or subtractions, learning new habits or skills, or compensating for a trauma such as the loss of a limb or a stroke.

If this concept seems strange, you are not alone. Most 20th-century neuroscientists believed that the brain was basically static after childhood development, and only recently have we realized how wrong we were. For example, a recent study showed that learning to juggle over a three month period stimulated significant physical growth in the areas of the brain associated with visual and motor function. And this is not a uni-directional phenomenon: those participants who gave up juggling entirely for another three months showed a return to their original brain size.[1] So the brain seems to be much more like a muscle than we knew. Both organs react and grow to accommodate the activities we pursue, and if we stop those activities then our muscles/brains atrophy in order not to waste energy maintaining physical or mental potential that we are not going to use.

So in just three months of moderate juggling practice, the brain is triggered by behavior to grow and change in ways meant to make juggling easier and more rewarding in the future. Now try to tally up how many hours over how many years regular porn users spend masturbating to pornography or to pornographic fantasy, digging porn-induced pathways into their brains that they now rely on for sexual gratification. A recent Cambridge study used an MRI (magnetic resonance imager) to scan the brains of healthy volunteers and self-reported compulsive pornography users as they were shown video clips of porn. The resulting images show in porn addicts very similar

---

[1] Jones, R. (2004, March). Juggling boosts the brain. *Nature Reviews Neuroscience*. Web.

changes to what occurs in an alcoholic's or a drug addict's brain: significantly stronger response in "the ventral striatum, which is [...] involved in processing reward, motivation and pleasure," indicating that their desires had been neurophysiologically conditioned for porn.[2]

Healthy
Volunteers

Compulsive
Pornography
Users

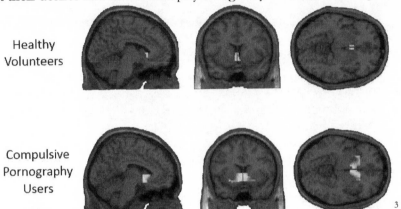

[3]

All addictions, whether to substances or behaviors, cause similar changes in the brain. Perhaps the most notable changes occur in the limbic system, which among other functions regulates desire and motivation. Habit-forming drugs like cocaine, opiates, nicotine, and alcohol are addictive because they interact with our brains' natural reward systems, hijacking mechanisms that naturally impel us toward beneficial goals and reward us with good feelings for achievement. Super-stimulating activities like viewing Internet porn, playing video games, or gambling can hijack these systems in similar ways because they cause unusually powerful changes in our brain's endogenous (built-in) neurochemicals. Any of these addictions results in a typical series of effects, including a rising tolerance for the substance or activity, an increasing craving for the addiction, and a reduction in the desire for and pleasure from natural rewards.[4]

How exactly these physical changes occur is complex, but according to Doctors Nestler and Malenka, experts on addiction and authors on neuropharmacology, they stem primarily from proteins

[2] Withnall, A. (2013, September 22). Pornography addiction leads to same brain activity as alcoholism or drug abuse, study shows. *The Independent*. Web.

[3] Voon, Valerie. *Porn on the Brain*. Channel 4.

[4] Nestler, E. (2005, October 26). Is there a common molecular pathway for addiction?. *Nature Neuroscience*.
http://www.nature.com/neuro/journal/v8/n11/full/nn1578.html

called "transcription factors" that activate genes and sculpt the long-term functionality of the brain and nervous system. One transcription factor, CREB, is responsible for building tolerance to a drug or stimulus, meaning that it takes a greater potency or quantity of the substance to produce the same feeling of pleasure. These effects can wear off relatively quickly, so an abstaining addict will be more sensitive to re-exposure than usual. Another strange-sounding transcription factor, Delta-FosB, sensitizes addiction pathways in the brain's reward system, causing the individual to have a heightened desire for his vice. Unlike CREB, Delta-FosB can remain active in the brain for months—even when the addict completely abstains. Recent research further suggests that physical brain changes and increased sensitivity caused by Delta-FosB can persist years after the protein itself has diminished, leaving addicts vulnerable to relapse long after they may consider themselves cured.[5]

Additionally, long-term addiction of any type has been shown to cause atrophy (weakening and shrinkage) in the frontal lobe of the brain. The frontal lobe contains the prefrontal cortex and is responsible for (among other things) reasoned planning, decision making, and self-restraint—in other words, willpower. Unsurprisingly, this lessened capacity for self-control serves to further perpetuate the addictive cycle. Originally demonstrated in drug addiction, "hypofrontality" has now been found to develop in behavioral addicts as well, as demonstrated by a 2011 Chinese study on Internet addicts.[6] Even more recently, a study out of Germany negatively associated hours viewing pornography each week with the amount of gray matter (brain cells) in the striatum, which coordinates motivation and action with higher-level logical thinking.[7] The functional connectivity between the striatum and the prefrontal cortex was also negatively associated with porn use.[8] In

---

[5] Nestler, E. J., & Malenka, R. C. (2004, March). The addicted brain. *Scientific American, 290*(3), 78-85.

[6] Yuan K, Qin W, Wang G, Zeng F, Zhao L, et al. (2011) Microstructure abnormalities in adolescents with Internet addiction disorder. PLoS ONE 6(6). Web.

[7] Rolls, E. (Aug–Sep 1994). Neurophysiology and cognitive functions of the striatum. *Révue Neurologique* 150 (8–9), 648–60.

[8] Kühn, S., Gallinat, J. (2014, May 28). Brain structure and functional connectivity associated with pornography consumption: The brain on porn. *JAMA Psychiatry*. Web.

other words, the higher the level of porn consumption, the weaker and less-functional the brain tends to be.

Why did the human brain evolve to make us so vulnerable to addiction? Simply put, transcription factors like CREB and Delta-FosB help to make us adaptive to our environment. CREB protects our brains from over stimulation, while Delta-FosB reinforces our desire to perform activities that are inherently rewarding, such as exercising, eating high-calorie foods, and having positive social interactions. Problems only arise when our brains' natural tools are responding to unnaturally powerful stimuli, such as mind-altering drugs, heavily processed foods, or hyper-stimulating Internet porn.

Recently more and more studies target the consistent computer and video game use that is so common in our information age, but there is not yet a wealth of peer-reviewed information specifically on the effects of consistent masturbation to high-speed Internet porn. This is partly because Internet porn addiction is a relatively new phenomenon: though pornography has been around for thousands of years, never before the 1990's has an unlimited amount of infinitely varied stimulation been available to the masses in the privacy of their own homes and with the ease of a few keystrokes. Another reason for the lack of research and recognition is that the negative effects of porn addiction are gradual and often not noticed until the man in question starts losing his erections or hears another man's story and relates it to his own problems. Third, the effects of porn addiction are by nature embarrassing, and most men do not freely discuss it. Finally, even when researchers realize the importance of this topic and attempt to study it, they are often stymied by the inability to form a control group, as it is extremely difficult to find young men who do not watch porn.

Now if you are like I was a short time ago, you probably scoff at my use of the words "addict" and "addiction" in relation to porn use. You are no junkie with a needle in his arm, and neither am I. No, what we have is a behavioral addiction. According to the article, "Diagnostic instruments for behavioral addiction: an overview", "The psychotropic effect [of a behavioral addiction] consists of the body's own biochemical processes induced only by excessive activities"[9], meaning that any activity that releases the right neurochemicals in our brains can

---

[9] Albrecht, U., Kirschner, N., & Grüsser, S. (2007, October 4). Diagnostic instruments for behavioural addiction: An overview. *National Center for Biotechnology Information*. Web.

become an addiction. These activities can include gambling, shopping, working, or unhealthy codependence, but people are particularly prone to become addicted to the behaviors that are most naturally rewarding, such as (over) eating and (compulsive) sexual activity.

Our brains are wired to binge eat when we encounter calorie-rich foods, a rare treat in the natural world that will help us survive until the next find. Of course, this neurological process becomes a problem when we have unlimited access to fatty, sugary foods, which is part of why obesity has become such a widespread problem in the developed world: we are wired to overindulge. But there is hope. We do not have to be slaves to this wiring. We do share the same basic limbic system with other animals, but we also boast a frontal lobe that is far more developed than in most creatures, allowing us greater control over our impulses. As detailed above, however, this control can be lessened by addiction-induced hypofrontality.

Similar to food, when we men (and to a lesser degree women) encounter several willing, attractive mates, we are wired to copulate with all of them, finding new thrill in the variety that cannot be found by having sex with the same mate repeatedly. This is known as the "Coolidge effect", a label that comes from an old joke about President Calvin Coolidge. The story goes that the President and Mrs. Coolidge were touring an experimental government farm. Mrs. Coolidge noticed that the rooster in the chicken yard was mating very frequently, so she asked how often the rooster mated and was told, "Dozens of times each day." The first lady nodded wryly and said, "Tell that to the President when he comes by." When the message was relayed, President Coolidge asked, "Same hen every time?" The attendant replied, "Oh no, Mr. President, a different hen every time. To which the President said, "Tell that to Mrs. Coolidge."[10]

Sooty the guinea pig became famous for demonstrating the Coolidge effect in south Wales in 2000, when Sooty escaped from his cage and tunneled into the female guinea pig enclosure. While the researchers scratched their heads as to where Sooty could have gone, over the next two days he copulated with all 24 females and later became the proud father of 42 guinea piglets. The researchers found Sooty exhausted in the corner of the female cage and returned him to

---

[10] Dewsbury, Donald A. (2000) *Portraits of Pioneers in Psychology, Volume 4*, (pp. 269-281).

his home, where he slept for two days recovering from his exertions.[11]

Such a desire to binge when we can allows us the best chance to pass on our genetic material, but watching Internet porn hijacks the natural reward circuits for sex, as the limbic system in our brains (the one responsible for recognizing reward and motivating pursuit) interprets an endless parade of porn stars as real novel mates, even though our cerebral cortex (the rational mind) knows better. After enough time, a single real mate just does not elicit as exciting of a dopamine kick as the porn does, and addiction takes root.

In this book I follow the American Society of Addiction Medicine's definition of addiction: "Addiction is a primary, chronic disease of brain reward, motivation, memory and related circuitry." This means that addiction itself is its own disorder, no matter the object of the addiction. ASAM's short definition of addiction continues, "Addiction is characterized by inability to consistently abstain, impairment in behavioral control, craving, diminished recognition of significant problems with one's behaviors and interpersonal relationships, and a dysfunctional emotional response. Like other chronic diseases, addiction often involves cycles of relapse and remission."[12] Notice that there is nothing about consistency of use in this definition. Contrary to what we might imagine when thinking of a porn addict, one does not have to use porn unusually often to be an addict.

Addiction is well studied, but addiction to Internet porn has only just begun to receive attention and is not yet recognized as an official disorder by the American Psychiatric Association (APA). If you are like me, though, you would rather not wait years for the psychiatric community to catch up with the facts of porn addiction in order to heal yourself. So let us start by defining a rubric for the presence and severity of addiction. The following 11 criteria are inspired by the APA's substance addiction diagnostic tool,[13] and with some adaptation each criterion applies equally as well to porn use (except maybe number eight, but who am I to judge?). You can also adapt these criteria to analyze any other addictive behavior, such as gambling, masturbation,

---

[11] Romeo guinea pig causes baby boom. (2000, November 30). *BBC News*. Web.

[12] Public policy statement: Definition of addiction. (2011, August 15). *American Society of Addiction Medicine*. Web.

[13] *Diagnostic and statistical manual of mental disorders: DSM-5*. (5th ed.). (2013). Substance use disorders (pp. 483, 484). Washington, D.C.: American Psychiatric Association.

etc. Make a tally mark for every statement that applies to you.

- 1: You use more extreme pornographic material than you planned, use porn more frequently than you planned, or have used porn over a greater time span than you planned.
- 2: You have several times expressed that you would like to quit or reduce use and/or have unsuccessfully tried to reduce or stop use.
- 3: You spend an inordinate or inconvenient amount of time acquiring, using, and/or recovering from the effects of porn.
- 4: You experience strong cravings for porn.
- 5: You have compromised major obligations at home, at work, or at school due to porn use.
- 6: You continue using porn despite knowing that it is consistently causing or worsening social or interpersonal problems.
- 7: You have skipped or given up significant social or occupational activities in order to use porn.
- 8: You use porn in ways or locations that are physically hazardous.
- 9: You continue using porn despite knowing that it is consistently causing or worsening physical or psychological problems.
- 10: You have acquired a tolerance and need more lengthy, varied, or extreme porn to feel the same or similar pleasure as when you first started using.
- 11: You experience unpleasant withdrawal symptoms when you abstain and may use porn to alleviate these symptoms.

According to the APA, "As a general estimate of severity, a *mild* substance use disorder is suggested by the presence of two to three symptoms, *moderate* by four to five symptoms, and *severe* by six or more symptoms."[14] If two or more of these criteria apply to you, then your porn use has likely escalated from pastime to problem. This book will give you the information necessary to decide if you want to fix that problem, as well as a detailed guide for how to do so. And if you are curious, I scored a nine.

Remember that this tool is not endorsed by the APA, and addiction to pornography is not yet recognized by the APA as a mental disorder. I only intend for these criteria to help you determine if porn use has become a problem in your life so that you can make an informed decision about using it in the future.

---

[14] *Diagnostic and statistical manual of mental disorders: DSM-5.* (5th ed.). (2013). Substance use disorders (pp. 484). Washington, D.C.: American Psychiatric Association.

She just doesn't do it for me (psychological and physiological symptoms)

By now you have a better idea of whether or not you or someone you know may be an (unofficial) addict. If you are, then PMO (porn, masturbation, orgasm) has likely affected your life in ways you never realized. Even if you do not self-identify as an addict or fulfill any of the above addiction criteria, however, you may still suffer from negative symptoms caused by over-consumption of porn. The following are the most common symptoms of compulsive PMO along with anecdotal information and descriptions of how these symptoms reverse after healing.

Porn-induced erectile dysfunction (PIED) and **reduced libido** especially tend to jolt men into researching their problems and discovering the connection between their sexual dysfunction and porn use. In 2000, Dr. Jennifer P. Schneider conducted a survey of nearly 100 partners of cybersex addicts. According to her results, "fully half of the 94 respondents (49, or 52.1%) said that their husbands were not interested, or hardly interested in sex with them."[15] If you are a porn-watching man (especially a young man) in generally good health who has lost interest in real sex or has difficulty "getting it up" or keeping it up with a partner, porn use is probably the cause.

Men often blame their reduced libido on their partners not being sexually attractive or adventurous enough, but it is near impossible for any lone woman to compete with the dopamine rush that a porn addict gets when using. PIED may manifest in copulatory impotence, in which the user can still perform just fine for the computer screen but wilts when the real deal comes along. Other heavy users may find it difficult to get hard even to porn and need to take a break in order to allow their tolerance to subside. It is also common to blame these problems on substance use (whiskey dick) or performance anxiety, and these can be factors. After all, who would not be anxious about his sexual performance after failing to perform several times? Plenty of

---

[15] Schneider, J. (2000). Effects of cybersex addiction on the family: Results of a survey. *jenniferschneider.com*. Web.

men throughout history have had sex just fine while stinking drunk, however, and the root cause is most likely consistent PMO.

Unlike in most older men with ED, the source of PIED is not in our clogged arteries or our penises but in our brains. During a session of Internet PMO, we likely encounter more willing, attractive mates (as interpreted by our limbic systems) in an hour than we would in a year without porn or other suggestive media. This is especially true if we use "compilation" videos and/or multiple windows and tabs rather than sitting down for a single VHS as our dads did. This results in something called "supranormal" stimulation. In short, this means that we are experiencing far more dopamine release than natural events would normally trigger, and we are experiencing it consistently. Because the brain is plastic, our reward circuitry adapts. The dopamine-sensitive neurons in the brain that are responsible for picking up the dopamine signal and translating it into pleasure and desire are overloaded. To protect themselves from overuse, these cells reduce the number of dopamine receptors available to receive dopamine.[16] On our next porn session, then, we are less sensitive to the same triggers. In order to reach a similar high, we need to find a way to release even more dopamine and fill every one of those reduced receptors that we can, so we escalate, finding more variety in the quantity and quality of the porn that we watch.

But the desensitization process that we triggered with porn and masturbation extends beyond those activities and into actual sex. Men with porn-induced ED find themselves less aroused by their partners, often needing to fantasize about extreme porn or to engage is porn-like, visually oriented sex just to maintain an erection. Often these men are very mentally attracted to their partners and very much want to have sex, but that desire does not translate into physical arousal.

Fortunately, with enough time away from porn this problem seems to solve itself.

Anonymous: *At 51, I went to the doctor seeking answers for my ED. He told me the same thing, "It's all in your head," after asking me a few questions about my sex life (nothing about porn use, though). Oh, I had blood work done a few months before that and my testosterone and other hormones were all in the normal range.*

He gave me a few samples of Viagra to "get my confidence back." But said he

---

[16] Nestler, E. (2005, October 26). Is there a common molecular pathway for addiction?. *Nature Neuroscience*. Web.

did not feel I needed to be on it as a regular medication. That was six months ago and my finding has been that it isn't just psychological. What I have learned from others on this forum, plus other articles on porn induced ED rings true. I'm a few days away from the 90 day mark (porn abstinence) and am seeing remarkable progress. Just slow dancing with my spouse gets me hot and bothered now. And my soldier salutes!

Porn-induced delayed ejaculation and **reduced sensitivity** can be precursors to or occur in conjunction with PIED, and their causes are much the same: desensitization due to porn use and masturbation. Men with PIDE complain of taking too long to orgasm with a partner or of the inability to orgasm without using their own hands. Aside from being desensitized neurochemically, these men are often desensitized to physical touch due to frequent masturbation and increasingly rough masturbation, i.e. "death grip". Like its neurochemical counterpart, physical sensitivity returns over time, though men with this problem often must cease masturbation altogether in order to re-sensitize.

Anonymous: *Listen to me. NoFap* [no masturbation] *worked for my severe case. Follow through. Don't edge. I've struggled with DE for 7 years...7 FUCKING YEARS. It ruined my confidence, my sanity, and it almost ruined my relationship.*

I've tested the theory 10+ times. Anytime I have a streak of NoFap and have sexual relations, I finish. Every time I'm off the wagon, I can't cum from anyone else's touch but my own. I refuse to live that way.

After having some perfect, mind-blowing sex this evening (and finishing), I can say with absolute certainty I'm never going back to fapping. This is it. Everything was just perfect tonight and I know it's because of NoFap.

Ironically, at the same time addicts may be experiencing desensitization, they have probably also been **sensitized to porn**. As detailed previously, this is in part due to transcription factors that hardwire heavily used reward pathways into the brain, increasing desire for porn even as the sensations of masturbating become less pleasurable. This reward sensitization is likely to persist long after the physical symptoms have been relieved, which is why former addicts are more susceptible to returning to compulsive use after re-exposure than is someone who has never been addicted. Imagine a year-long sober alcoholic suddenly diving back into a bender after experiencing a tragedy—or a man who has been porn-free for months binging for hours on his computer after convincing himself that he was cured and could watch borderline material without relapsing. Consider the following PMO addict.

Never2Fap: *Well, looks like I made the 90 days without even one relapse. I came close a few times but I always conquered myself with willpower. I'm a much stronger man now than I was back in November 2013 and I will not be picking the fapping back up. Keep up the hard work, don't give up, and yes it's definitely worth it.*

(Several months later)

I have failed. Not just a little bit, but to the utmost extreme, going back to my old ways in every way for 3 months straight. Wanting to quit, wondering what went wrong. What a sad sack of burning hell my life has become in 3 months of abuse. Today I vow to start anew!

I know what went wrong, I got lazy and weak. I lied to myself and made excuses about why a little use and abuse was okay here and there. How a fap every month might be good for you, then it became once a week, then it happened out of my control.

I'm sorry guys, I've disappointed myself and failed. I'm coming back today.

In some men, porn use actually increases penile sensitivity and causes them to orgasm very quickly with a partner, which can be just as embarrassing and damaging to sexual confidence as PIED or PIDE. **Porn-induced premature ejaculation**, as it is called, claims a minority of reported porn-induced sexual dysfunction cases. However, many more young men (18-59) experience PE than ED,[17] and it is possible that a significant percentage of these cases are unknowingly caused by PMO dependence. Fortunately, the same healing process that cures PIED and PIDE can also alleviate PIPE, which comes in varied forms.

Anonymous: *So many men here at YBR and YBOP have "porn induced" Erectile Dysfunction (ED) and Delayed Ejaculation (DE). But some of us (I believe a minority) have premature ejaculation (PE) from our porn use.*

Prior to my reboot, my penis would get so rock hard and stand at attention at 12 o'clock. the skin on my penis stretched tight like a snare drum. My penis was a fueled up rocket sitting on the launch pad, countdown starts at 10 seconds, 9, 8, 7, 6,5,4,3,2,1…ORGASM. The words "sorry honey" became my motto.

But today, 52 days into re-boot, my penis is no longer on the rocket launch pad. It stands at 10 O'clock. I have a softer, but bigger erection. Don't get me wrong, It is still very hard and capable of V penetration. It is more plastic now and less rigid. It is less sensitive, not ready to explode. But most important to my relationship with my wife, I am able to last longer now. The reboot is working very well on my porn-induced PE!

---

[17] Castleman, M. (2010, May 28). Premature Ejaculation: The Two Causes of Men's #1 Sex Problem. *Psychology Today*. Web.

Other men experience a combination of PIED and PIPE; they achieve erection only with difficulty but then ejaculate very quickly—the worst of both worlds.

Anonymous: *I seem to suffer from both ED and premature ejaculation. When I would begin to get it on with a lady once I had an erection I would ejaculate very quickly (like 10-15 sec). I'm on the NoFap wagon to hopefully eliminate the ED but I'm not so sure about the premature ejaculation. When I did masturbate it would be bedtime so I would try to finish as quickly as possible so I could go to sleep. I think this coupled with nervousness with a girl is what is ultimately responsible for the premature ejaculation.*

Some even begin to ejaculate without ever achieving erection.

Anonymous: *Some of us are initially faced with an awful choice: Erectile Dysfunction or Premature Ejaculation. In fact, I had both at the same time. That was my low point during recovery. It wouldn't get hard just making out, so she touched it (soft) and it exploded (soft). This, for me anyway, was a temporary condition. Once I was able to get hard regularly (and I thankfully have a willing partner) and was able to have sex on a frequent enough basis, I now get hard quickly and easily AND stay hard long enough for her to be completely satisfied.*

There are several theories as to why PE develops in some porn users—none of them scientifically tested. Some testify that for years they tried to climax as quickly as possible during PMO, either to avoid getting caught or because they wanted quick relief without wasting too much time. Gradually they trained their bodies to orgasm quickly with minimal stimulation. Similarly, some men begin lose erections during masturbation to porn but still want the rush of ejaculation, so they push through to orgasm regardless. Either of these habits can become ingrained behaviors and carry over into sex with a partner.

Tolerance is a medical term that describes the decrease over time in the body's response to a stimulus, necessitating a greater quality or quantity to achieve the same result. For example, an alcoholic who can down five drinks and barely show it—or a porn user who has lost interest in risqué magazines and moved on to hardcore streaming videos. As a defense mechanism, the body builds a resistance, or tolerance, against whatever substance is causing dramatic changes in the body, including an unusually high and consistent release of the brain's own dopamine supply. However, the user still wants to achieve the same high, so he increases the intensity of his chosen vice.

In porn addicts, tolerance leads to an **escalation** in the quantity or kinds of material users seek out. Men commonly start with nude pictures, escalate to videos of solo women, lesbians, or straight sex (this of course varies among non-heterosexual men), escalate again to anal and oral sex, and continue to escalate into whatever porn genres most excite them. Eventually, this can become a problem when men are getting off to subjects that actually disgust them and make them doubt their own sexuality. They are excited by these stimuli while masturbating but often immediately feel guilt and disgust after orgasm, wondering why they are turned on by porn featuring rough/violent sex, extreme submission and/or domination, transsexuals, urine, scat, bestiality, incest, or other unusual and extreme elements. The answer is that it is easier in a desensitized brain to reach the heights of sexual excitement when lust is paired with another primal emotion in the right conditions, such as anger, fear, shock, disgust, or shame.

Never2Fap: *In these 100 days the #1 thing I've found to have changed that I am most thankful for is the fact that I no longer like disgusting abuse porn. When I was addicted to PMO I would seek out the most deviant sites I could find and I didn't care who the girls were or what they were going through. [...] The addiction was stronger than I thought, and it was twisting and controlling my mind.*

Now after just 100 days I'm clean. I love women instead of lust them. I want to see happy women with fulfilled lives. I want to see their faces and their curves. I want to see their eyes sparkling and know that they are going home and sleeping happily at night with a loving husband, just like my wife does. I don't even have the desire to look at porn anymore. I have my wife and she is more than enough for me. If I didn't have her, I'd be looking for her.

Because these men are no longer sufficiently aroused by simple nude men or women or vanilla sex, they may understandably begin to doubt their sexual orientation, confused by the subjects they find themselves masturbating to. This is especially true when straight men start viewing transsexual or homosexual porn or homosexual men start viewing heterosexual or lesbian porn, which can lead to **sexual orientation obsessive compulsive disorder**, a condition characterized by fear of actually being homosexual or heterosexual when the opposite feels natural and right. A heterosexual man who has escalated in his porn use may feel excited by a clip of gay porn, which causes him to fear that he has homosexual tendencies. The more he fears this possibility, the more he tests himself by looking at other men and viewing homosexual porn, developing H(homosexual)OCD in the process. HOCD, however, does not stem from natural sexual tendencies but rather from fear and insecurity. Often men with porn-induced HOCD find that by giving up porn, they return to being aroused by real women and vanilla sex, and the fear slips away.

Emotional numbness is one of the more gradual and difficult-to-recognize symptoms of consistent PMO. Just as desensitization to porn bleeds over into actual sex, so too does it extend into the rest of addicts' lives, as dopamine and other related neurochemicals play a strong role in much more than just sexual arousal and response. Many porn addicts use PMO to relieve themselves of difficult emotions like loneliness and stress, but what they do not realize is that we cannot numb the bad without numbing the good as well, and all of life gets a little more gray. This change only really becomes apparent once addicts cease PMO and their lost emotional landscapes begin to reassert themselves.

Anonymous: *What most people don't seem to be acknowledging is that you will encounter emotions you haven't felt for years, maybe never. Girls that didn't matter to you before will all of a sudden be the centerpiece to your f—king life. That test you failed? You don't blow it off; you worry about your grade; you worry about the final coming up in two weeks. And this is good; hell it's great. This is the suffering that you learn from, that grows you as a person. But it will hurt. At points you'll feel sad, confused, maybe even depressed. But don't fall into that trap. Emotions pass, memories fade, and you will come out stronger for it. Remember, you have years of emotional growth and maturity to come into. It might not be easy, you may not feel comfortable, but it is worth it.*

Social anxiety, depression, apathy, and "brain fog" are often ameliorated or even alleviated by ceasing PMO. Wilson cites several articles that may explain why this happens. One study published in 2002 examines the relationship between social rank, dopamine receptors, and vulnerability to cocaine addiction among a group of cynomolgus macaques (monkeys).[18] Bear with me.

Socially dominant monkeys displayed more acts of aggression than subordinates (average 1.9 vs. 0 episodes/hour), were submitted to more often (3.0 vs. 0.1 episodes/hour), were groomed more often (12.1% vs. 4.9% of the time), and spent significantly less time alone (14.8% vs. 27.8%). The subordinate monkeys, on the other hand, submitted often, displayed little aggression, and enjoyed less social capital.

Researchers on this study discovered that, when housed alone, all 20 monkeys had about the same amount of dopamine D_2 receptors.

---

[18] Morgan, D., Grant, K., Gage, H., Mach, R., Prioleau, O., Nader, S., et al. (2002, February). Social dominance in monkeys: Dopamine D2 receptors and cocaine self-administration. *National Center for Biotechnology Information*. Web.

After three months of living together, however, those monkeys who had established themselves as dominant showed an increase in D_2 receptors of more than 20%, while the subordinate monkeys displayed no significant change, indicating that the dominant monkeys' social behavior had effected this neurophysiologic difference.

Then the researchers gave the monkeys controlled access to cocaine, discovering that the dominant monkeys with more D_2 receptors were significantly less vulnerable to cocaine dependency than their subordinates. Since interviews were impossible, it is hard to know why the D_2 receptor-rich monkeys were less interested in cocaine, but I like to think that the cool, confident monkeys found enough satisfaction in real life that artificial pleasure paled in comparison.

You may wonder: if it was the dominant behavior that triggered the rise in D_2 receptors and not the other way around, what good are the receptors? It is likely, though, that dominant behavior and D_2 receptors create a positive feedback loop with one another, as dominant behavior increases D_2 receptors and a greater amount of D_2 receptors have been shown to cause a rise in desirable and dominant traits, such as motivation and attention span[19] as well as resistance to drug addiction.[20] Indeed, when the D_2 concentration of all monkeys are chemically reduced to equal levels, the social hierarchy dissolves.[21] Though similar tests cannot ethically be performed on humans, a 2010 study showed that people who enjoy higher social status and increased levels of social support also display a higher density of dopamine D_2 receptors, while a lower density is associated with lower social status and decreased social support.[22]

What does all of this mean for us porn addicts? Well, in humans

---

[19] Trifilieff, P., Feng, B., Urizar, E., Winiger, V., Ward, R., Taylor, K., et al. (2013, September). Increasing dopamine D2 receptor expression in the adult nucleus accumbens enhances motivation. *nature.com*. Web.

[20] DOE/Brookhaven National Laboratory. (2008, April 18). Gene therapy for addiction: Flooding brain with 'pleasure chemical' receptors works on cocaine, as on alcohol. *ScienceDaily*. Web.

[21] Czoty, P., Morgan, D., Shannon, E., Gage, H., Nader, M.. (2004, July). Characterization of dopamine D1 and D2 receptor function in socially housed cynomolgus monkeys self-administering cocaine. *National Center for Biotechnology Information*. Web.

[22] Elsevier. (2010, February 7). Brain dopamine receptor density correlates with social status. *ScienceDaily*. Web.

low levels of D_2 receptors have been associated with ADHD,[23] low motivation,[24] social anxiety,[25] and conditioned fear.[26] In 2005 a high-functioning, healthy medical student demonstrated these relationships when he volunteered to have his dopamine levels chemically stunted. The result: he experienced loss of concentration, memory, motivation, and vocal fluency as well as increased tiredness, shame, fear, anxiety, and depression.[27] So when we force our limbic systems to desensitize with repeated porn-induced dopamine spikes, we may be making ourselves less confident, determined, and attentive and more fearful and addiction-prone—in pack terms, "beta". Not exactly the qualities most of us strive for. Ultimately, this may help to explain why, as a recovering porn addict's brain re-sensitizes by activating more dopamine receptors, he often also experiences greater confidence, focus, motivation, energy, emotional depth, and social ability.

Anonymous: *For years I've had social anxiety, suffered from depression, no motivation...I had some social contact but it was mostly superficial. I didn't really bother getting to know people. Nothing interested me, I just went from day to day not really doing anything. But worst of all, looking back, was that I was I was generally unhappy and didn't really care that I was. I guess you could say the world was black and white.*

But now, for the first time in several years, I'm looking forward to the new year. I feel...happy, for several reasons. I've met new people, and got to know stuff about them. I'm genuinely interested in them. I can focus on my studies better, sort of remembering why I started them in the first place. I picked up my guitar, and I'm

[23] Volkow, N., Wang, G., Kollins, S., Wigal, T., Newcorn, J., Telang, F., et al. (2009, September 9). Evaluating dopamine reward pathway in ADHD. *National Center for Biotechnology Information*. Web.

[24] Volkow, N., Wang, G., Newcorn, J., Kollins, S., Wigal, T., Telang, F., et al. (2010, September 21). Motivation Deficit in ADHD is Associated with Dysfunction of the Dopamine Reward Pathway. *National Center for Biotechnology Information*. Web.

[25] Schneier, F., Liebowitz, M., Abi-Dargham, A., Zea-Ponce, Y., Lin, S., Laruelle, M.(2000, March). Low dopamine D2 receptor binding potential in social phobia. *American Journal of Psychiatry*, 157(3), 457-459.

[26] Oliveira, A. d., Reimer, A., Macedo, C. d., Carvalho, M. d., Silva, M., & Brandão, M. (2011, January). Conditioned fear is modulated by D2 receptor pathway connecting the ventral tegmental area and basolateral amygdala. *National Center for Biotechnology Information*. Web.

[27] Haan, L., Booij, J., Lavalye, J., Amelsvoort, T., Linszen, D. (2005 September).Subjective experiences during dopamine depletion. *American Journal of Psychiatry*, 162(9), 1755-1755.

learning Spanish.

The world isn't a black and white place anymore. There are colours now, and they're awesome! Sure, I may not have access to the full colour palette yet, but I'm willing to keep painting. Not all my problems were PMO related, but I guess it was the last drop in the bucket. Removing the drop helped me to work on myself.

Impaired sleep is another symptom that may only become apparent retrospectively as it improves over time, and this symptom may surprise many users who in fact use PMO as a way to fall asleep. This works because orgasm releases a whole slew of neurochemicals into the nervous system that result in tiredness, but a 2012 study shows that dopamine activity—such as that encountered during PMO— actually interferes with the body's synthesis of melatonin, a hormone that plays a key role in regulating the sleep-wake cycle.[28] So while after orgasm we may be able to fall asleep just fine, the quality of that sleep and our ability to wake up refreshed and alert in the morning may be impaired. Recovering addicts often report more vivid dreams and changes in sleep patterns, though for those who rely on PMO to sleep, interrupting that habit is likely to make their rest worse before it gets better.

Reduced athletic performance and muscle mass is a symptom reported anecdotally but is thus far untested by the scientific community. In fact—and contrary to traditional thinking—recent research shows that orgasm the night before a sporting event does not actually reduce athletic performance.[29] But there is no study concerning the long-term effects of chronic PMO on physicality and athleticism. Like with sleep quality, many men only notice after they quit that their cardiovascular endurance, strength, and muscle mass have been suppressed. These changes can be partly explained by the increased motivation and free time to pursue fitness, but some men insist that PMO itself was a major negative influence on their athleticism.

---

[28] González, S., Moreno-Delgado, D., Moreno, E., Pérez-Capote, K., Franco, R., et al. (2012) Circadian-related heteromerization of adrenergic and dopamine D_4 receptors modulates melatonin synthesis and release in the pineal gland. *PLoS Biology*. Web.

[29] Sztajzel, J., Périat, M., Marti, V., Krall, P., & Rutischauser, W. (2000, September). Effect of sexual activity on cycle ergometer stress test parameters, on plasmatic testosterone levels and on concentration capacity. A study in high-level male athletes performed in the laboratory. *National Center for Biotechnology Information*. Web.

Similarly, **a wasted appearance and acne** are also often self-reported by PMO addicts who have improved their appearance with abstinence from porn and masturbation, but no studies yet attempt to link the two.

Anonymous: *I was spending 3 or 4 hours every single day "trying to find that next perfect girl" and busting my nut once almost every single day. I started to get tired all the time, my face was becoming pale, these dark circles were formed under my eyes constantly, I was sleeping 10 hours a day and STILL waking up tired, AND I began pulling clumps & clumps of hair out of the shower. I remember my old girls I used to hook up with would meet me out at a bar or something and they would always have this shocked look on their face. "OMG is that him????" My other friends and family also commented on how skinny I was getting and I "need to eat more"...the funny thing was, I was a bodybuilder. I went from 220 to 180, no shit, even WITH exercising and eating lots of organic food and excess calories. I was whittling away to nothing. I started getting all these weird irrational fears around people. I felt shaky and weak. My voice is more hollow, if that makes sense. I lost myself. I was depressed constantly. I stopped leaving my house. My friends slowly faded. So I'm now a balding and skinny socially awkward pale weirdo, lol, where I used to be the King of my campus...wtf! I'm convinced, through irrefutable experience that this horrible shit is so fucking unnatural and drains a man's SOUL. I didn't change ANY OTHER VARIABLE IN MY LIFE except for getting addicted to pornography and fapping more often. That's it. I was still thinking positively, going out to bars, eating healthy, exercising, all that jazz. The ONLY thing that increased was my love affair with the fake girls on the blaring pixelated screen.*

Anonymous: *Wow, just wow. My skin has not looked this good in almost a year! I honestly do not know what to say except that it must be NoFap. My habits are the same, I am eating the same foods, I am drinking the same amount of water, exercising the same, working the same, same stress level, just NoFap! I strongly recommend anybody with acne to try NoFap, my skin actually looks GOOD now. I don't know exactly what it is in the NoFap, but there is something, whether it's raising or lowering hormones, testosterone, stress, whatever it is, NoFap works. I could not be happier with the results.*

It may seem incredible that all of these symptoms can be brought about only by frequent masturbation to pornography, but consider the reality that our nervous systems evolved to handle. For hundreds of thousands of years *Homo sapiens* and their ancestors lived in tribal societies in which there was a very limited selection of mates, so meeting a new attractive man or woman was a rarity that our limbic systems evolved to respond powerfully to. A situation in which several or many new attractive mates were present and willing was so rare an opportunity that our limbic systems would kick into overdrive, pushing us to copulate with all of them in order to pass on our genetic material.

The tachometer of a car measures how fast the engine is spinning so that we can shift gears appropriately. On the tachometer, a red line shows us the point at which we risk damaging the engine from running it too fast. Pushing into this range is not something you want to do if you can avoid it, but you would put the pedal to the floor anyway if you had the proper motivation. When our "binge drive" is activated by the imminent equivalent of winning the sex lottery, we push past our own red lines in order to fulfill our most important biological mission: to reproduce as much as possible. After all, we can always rest later, but such a sexual goldmine is rare and must be exploited now! Fortunately we are well equipped to handle and recover from this extra stress, so redlining on occasion is no big deal.

Fast-forward to the 21st century, when Internet pornography has been designed to hijack this binge drive by feeding our brains a constantly refreshing selection of extremely attractive mates doing anything we could ever want or imagine. Like Sooty the guinea pig after tunneling into the female cage or like the tribesman presented with a whole calendar's worth of Playmates, we want them all. But unlike Sooty or the tribesman, there is no end to our binge. That "later" in which we rest and recover from our sexual buffet need never come, because there is always more Internet porn to masturbate to. With porn, we activate a biological response that was designed to make us push past our normal limits—a response that in real life is activated only rarely but with porn can be exploited as often as we want, like pushing an engine past the red line day after day and never seeing a mechanic. It is no wonder that we are experiencing negative consequences.

My story

Once I decided to confront my own reliance on porn, I felt compelled to write it all down—all of my most private, painful, and joyous thoughts and memories concerning sex and love. I decided to share it with an anonymous online community called Your Brain Rebalanced. At 10,000 words, it contained a complete account of my sexual and romantic history—or at least the important bits. For those who want all the details, my entire post along with my following journal entries can still be found there under my pseudonym, "Spangler", but here I share just the parts of that story that I think will best help people understand porn addiction. The following was written at the beginning of my journey to recovery in January, 2014. Instead of summarizing my story from a current perspective, by using these words I choose to provide the most truthful representation of myself at that time.

As far back as I can remember (probably age 2-3) I have had a deep hunger for women that I satisfied with masturbation. For most of my childhood I didn't exactly whack it, just rubbed myself face down on the bed until climax each night (though of course there was no ejaculation at that time). I remember having vivid fantasies about the girls in preschool, women on TV, etc., and I never gave my nighttime (and occasionally daytime) habit much thought.

Sex was something of a taboo for me because of my parents, who seemed utterly sexless. I can count the number of times I've seen them kiss on one hand with room to spare, and they often didn't even sleep in the same room. When a romantic or sexual scene came onto the TV, my mother would sometimes tell me to look away or otherwise express disapproval. As I got older I voluntarily looked away, not because I wasn't interested in it but because I was embarrassed for her to know my interest. As an adult I would confront her about this, and she said it wasn't sex she disapproved of but rather raunchy behavior or the sexualization of women. At that age, however, I had no way to differentiate the "good" romance/sex from the "bad". My father was often absent and when present was a pillar of strength and the disciplinarian of the two, and bringing up my questions about sex with either of them was so out of my comfort zone that it didn't even seem an option. I want to be clear here: my parents were loving and nurturing and generally great parents, and I love them dearly to this day and forever. But they had absolutely no idea how to guide and teach a sex-driven boy—especially one in the electronic age. Thus I got my sexual education from Internet porn.

Up until this point I lived a vivid and rich sexual life in my imagination and still masturbated nightly, thinking mostly about girls in my life: undressing them, exploring their bodies—sometimes more than one at a time and in different settings. I thought about how my penis and the space between their legs would come together, but I didn't know what that space looked like and just imagined smooth skin.

We had a computer, and one day I had the idea to type "naked" into the picture search engine. Boom. I was hooked. I was 9 or 10. I would rub myself through my pants to the pictures and erotic stories, listening for footsteps and glancing around constantly so I could close the page at a moment's notice, then running upstairs to finish on my bed like usual. Of course, I didn't stop at naked pictures. Someone showed me how to download music illegally with programs like Kazaa, and it didn't take me long to figure out that you could download videos too.

Over the next 8 years I got deeper and deeper into porn, but I only was really able to indulge around age 13 when we moved and I got a computer in my room. I was definitely an addict. Don't get me wrong, I had school and friends and a life outside of my room, and I never had to "get my fix" at school or play pocket pool at the lunch table or anything like that, but porn was a consistent and exciting part of my life, and it obviously satisfied me enough that I didn't need to overcome my social anxiety in order to pursue real girls. The girls who flirted with me I didn't know how to handle, and because I had porn I didn't feel the need to figure it out. *I can always have real sex later*, I rationalized. *Besides, I'd really like to get home and read more of that story about the teenager with the harem.* It's not that I didn't want real sex, it's just that it was so much harder and more confusing to pursue than pornography. And romance wasn't the only part of my life I supplemented with technology. Video games, TV, and movies gradually replaced real-life adventure and experience.

But that wasn't enough for me forever. (Not, unfortunately, for my own personal satisfaction, but rather because as a male the social pressure to lose your virginity before graduation at the very latest was immense.) By the last two years in high school I had begun to get more involved in clubs and activities at school, and my social ability and self-confidence was rising. Somewhere along the line my cavalier facade and budding dry sense of humor attracted a certain pretty girl, who began messaging me over Google's chat. Cassandra. She asked me to homecoming dance, and I accepted. Though I was pretty nervous "IRL" I was able to sound smooth in text. Over the next weeks we flirted with and confided in each other through our Internet buffer, telling each other secrets and being sexually aggressive in a way we didn't have the courage to do in person. I'm looking back at this first conversation now, and there are 80 other separate conversations with her catalogued from over the next year in this old Gmail address (Google never deletes anything). Reading it now I'm cracking up at our suggestive innuendo, but I also see that I lied to her. She asked if I'd ever been in a sexual relationship, and I answered, "a couple", I guess rationalizing that kissing and holding hands during childhood was sexual in a way. I didn't want her to think less of me for being inexperienced. How destructive and damaging that thought process is.

When we finally went to homecoming, it went OK and horribly at the same time. I was planning for two whole days beforehand how I would kiss her, and I kept revising those plans up until and through the dance, and then the moment was gone and we hugged goodnight. I agonized over how I could have done better, and by the next day I was determined. I walked her to her car after school, and as the moment came to say goodbye I stood close to her, looked down into her eyes, and said, "There's something I wish I'd done last night." I leaned slowly into her and kissed a woman for the first time in about a decade. It was soft, sweet, and the perfect length for a first kiss. As I came out of it, I smiled slowly and said, "Goodbye." I then turned and walked steadily toward my car, not looking back for fear she'd see the huge grin on my face. I'll never forget that feeling. It was incredible, like a surge of life from deep inside me that pulsed into every tip and crevice of my body and mind. I'd never felt better about myself, and I laughed and cheered the whole drive home.

I had fantasies about how we would get closer and closer throughout the year, and that by the end of our high school career we would be lovers. This didn't happen. I'd led her to think that I was more experienced than I really was because of some false sense of pride, and I believe she was looking for someone like that to guide her. Of course, I was badly in need of guidance myself. We kissed a couple more times, but she grew more and more distant over time, and by December I was looking for other women.

Amy. She was two years younger than me but only a year beneath me in school. I wasn't as attracted to her as to Cassandra, but I could tell that she liked me very much. It felt good to be the one wanted, the one with more power. And besides, that virgin deadline was approaching, and if I still had my V-card when I went to college I would be among the lowest class of men there. I'm ashamed to say that this was a factor in starting our relationship. On Valentine's Day, I walked her to her bus and stood close, saying, "I have a Valentine's gift for you."

"What?" she asked, all big eyes and trembling expectations. I kissed her, deep but soft, and she let out a light moan into my mouth. "Happy Valentine's Day," I said, leaning back and looking her in the eyes. Then I left. I felt good. It wasn't the bursting, heart-pounding joy I had gotten from my first kiss with Cassandra; rather, it was more of a resounding masculine satisfaction. It definitely felt good. Later that evening, I saw she posted to Facebook that she'd never been so happy. (Or something to that effect. Looking at her FB now, it seems like everything from that year has been deleted or timed out, and her posts start in 2009.)

Some little time later we were alone in her house, necking on the common room couch and soon naked from the waist up. It was the first time I had been free to explore a woman's body, and I found her shoulders, neck, breasts, nipples, stomach—everything—fascinating. I noticed something strange, however. It was like I was detached, seeing myself from outside myself and directing my body from far away to do the things that I had read on the Internet would make her feel good. I also noticed that my penis did not react at all. *Huh,* I thought, *must just be because I'm not used to this and nervous.* But looking back, I wasn't really nervous. And I definitely found Amy attractive emotionally and physically. She said that this was as far as she wanted to go today, and—worried that I wouldn't be able to perform—I was glad of it.

The next time, we were in her bed. And the many times after that. I saw and felt and smelled her sex for the first time, and I did my best to please her with my fingers and my mouth. She wanted me to take her virginity, and I wanted it too, but my body seemed to disagree. I would get hard, but when the time came for penetration or putting the condom on I would go soft again. I recently found out from communities like this one that this is a common affliction among porn addicts, whose brains have become wired to respond only to constantly changing and stimulating clips. At the time though, I had no idea why it was happening. I thought I was broken. I thought I had been a virgin for too long and could no longer be comfortable reaching climax with anyone but myself. This was the most frustrating experience of my life till then, and it happened many times. Driving home from Amy's house, I would literally roar and beat the steering wheel with my fists in tortured anger. My biggest regret from this time, though, is that I never had the balls to just have an honest conversation with my girlfriend. She must have known that I couldn't talk about it, because all she said on the subject was, "It's okay." It did occur to me that maybe it was because I masturbated too often, so I stopped masturbating several days before seeing her. That didn't help, so I assumed it must just be that I had been so long alone that I couldn't yet be comfortable enough with a woman to achieve and maintain erection. I didn't know then that it can take months of abstinence from porn and masturbation to reboot your brain and open up/strengthen those original pathways that react to real women rather than increasingly extreme pixels.

The year was coming to a close. At our beginning, I had told her that I could not commit to her past graduation, because while I was leaving for college she had another year of high school, and I did not want a long-distance relationship (read: I wanted to gain some sexual experience with her and end it amicably so I could sleep around in college with confidence). At the time she agreed. Of course, emotions get messy. Or at least they do if you're not damaged in the way I was. She started to tell me that she loved me, and I started to say it back. *Maybe I do love her*, I rationalized. *I sure am fond of her—maybe that feeling is love.* However, when she began saying things like, "Never leave me," I realized that *Nope. Nope I am definitely not in love because that scares the living hell out of me.* I think I said in return, "I'll always be there for you," meaning, of course, *Sure I'll talk to you over chat sometimes between other women in college.*

Yet another effect of porn addiction: emotional numbness and inability to connect/empathize with others, especially women. I should note that I had not cried in about eight years at this time. Only right now as I am writing these words do I realize that this timing correlates almost exactly with when I got into porn. I also had felt hardly any extreme emotions but lust and anger in all that time. Mostly I coasted through my days getting good grades out of habit. I do not know how much of this apathy was due to pornography and how much can be put down to being a "normal" angsty teenager, but from the similar stories I've read from other porn addicts, I'm willing to bet that most of these emotional issues were due to my addiction.

My own rabid sexual insecurity at this point combined with a repulsion for Amy's need for me to effectively end our relationship. I became silent and moody around her, though I was still able to laugh and joke with other friends. When she understandably confronted me about it, I told her that graduation was coming and we would need to separate. I reminded her that I had warned her of this. She protested that she thought things had changed, or that at the least we would have the summer. At this point, though, I was so disgusted with my sexual failures that I couldn't be around her (not that I told her this, of course). She took it hard. She reached out to me several times and I listened to her cry on the other end of the phone. Mostly I just felt numb. I knew I should be more upset about this or caring for her, but I wasn't.

I should note here that porn addiction is not just for deviants and troublemakers. I was selected as one of 5 valedictorians for a class of 400. They chose the five students with the top weighted GPA's, though I was the only one who had never gotten anything but an A (no minuses). I say this not to brag but to show that the signs of an addiction like this aren't always reflected quantitatively in poor grades or detention slips. At graduation I spoke in front of more than 3500 people, and some pride and joy did shine through from this; my emotions hadn't completely flat-lined, just dulled—especially with women and relationships.

A couple weeks after graduation, Amy contacted me again. She had become violently ill with uncontrollable vomiting, pain, and other symptoms. She'd been to a doctor. She had breast cancer.

God.

Mostly what I felt at this time was a dull shock. I know what you're thinking. No way porn could have made him cold enough to shrug her off after this, right?

Well, you're right. I wasn't *that* much of an asshole. I was there to talk with her—like I promised, I suppose—and I spoke with her several times over the coming weeks during her treatment and recovery. I was mostly a brick wall, though. I couldn't even cry for this (or my grandfather's death, which occurred around this time), and all of my consolations sounded hollow in my own ears. I never saw her in person, and I haven't seen or talked with her since. Wait, that's not true...In college, I Skyped with her a small number of times. I don't remember much about it except that the conversations were lighthearted, and I flirted with her and sexualized her even though I certainly didn't deserve to. She seemed to enjoy it though. Maybe she needed to feel that I was still attracted to her. We haven't spoken since then...I'm pretty sure. According to Facebook she's got a boyfriend and a modeling career in Los Angeles.

Amy (though that's not your real name), if you ever read this, I am so sorry. I tried to use you and then when I couldn't even do that I discarded you. Know that I did have genuine affection for you and cherish many of the moments we shared and never wanted to hurt you. Know that I had unwittingly broken myself emotionally and sexually with my consistent porn use. At the same time your sickness almost took your life, my sickness robbed you of someone you thought you could trust, and I realize this now. I am sorry, and I wish you all the best.

Whew, OK. College. I basically regressed socially as my confidence was crippled by my impotence. I pursued several girls freshman year but was rejected by all (I don't blame them as at that time I was awkward as ****, partly from inexperience and party because of my porn-distorted view of human connection). I sunk deeper into electronic substitutes for life. After discovering that I could illegally pirate any movie with torrents and a high-speed Internet connection, I spent much of my free time watching movies, playing video games or pool with my roommate (who had a long-distance girlfriend), or masturbating to porn. Woohoo college.

I progressed slowly over the next year, but there was progress. I joined more activities, made more friends, and started drinking and partying. By sophomore year I had reconstructed my confidence well enough to attract and date another very beautiful woman. That said, nothing had changed for me sexually. And when it came to confronting this issue it gets even worse: I. Had. Learned. Nothing.

Yup. When I wasn't able to perform, I did not talk about it. I would try to please her in other ways for awhile and then I would pretend to be tired and go to sleep, but I actually lay awake torturing myself trying to find out why this was happening. She asked me if I'd had sex before, and I said, "Yes", rationalizing that a partial soft insertion must count, *right?* HA! My insecurities and rationalizations seem laughable now, which I guess is a good thing. Anyway, she was patient, but we never talked about it, and of course all the good times outside the bedroom can't really make up for a total, weighty, oppressive flop in the bedroom, so she ended it with me.

After that, there were other women, but I never progressed to the bed again until senior year of college. A semester abroad had given me many new friends, experiences, stories, and a much-needed boost of confidence by the time I returned to my home university. But I still could not ask for help. I had an overpowering need to be seen—and to see myself—as a pillar of masculinity. I could not reconcile that need with admitting my inexperience and difficulties. Instead, I tried to have sex, and when I couldn't make it work I would say that I wasn't ready to have sex with them. True enough, but not the whole truth. Though to be fair I didn't know the whole truth at that time either.

The previous summer I thought I had found out what the root of my problem was. I still believe that it is a big part of a lot of pain I have, but I do not anymore believe that it is the deciding cause of my total inability to be intimate (emotionally or physically) with a woman. The thing I'm talking about is circumcision. Four years previous, I got curious about circumcision and looked it up online. I was circumcised as an infant. When I got to the information about the negative effects of circumcision, I read for awhile and then closed my computer and put it out of my mind. It is the only time I can think of in my life when I chose ignorance over knowledge. I think I sensed something very painful down that road, and I avoided it. Well, I was right. That summer before Dalia, I was frustrated enough with my sexual issues that I decided to learn what I could about how circumcision had affected my life, and I found out that circumcision removes a lot of the nerve tissue in the penis, which in turn removes a lot of the possible sensations of sex.

Upon learning this and much more, I was horrified. I felt mutilated and betrayed. It seemed very likely that this was at least one cause of my sexual problems, as manual and oral stimulation from women felt much less amazing than I knew it should, and it was not enough for me to finish. But this is not a book about circumcision, so I'll leave out most of this part of my story, except for how it relates to my decision to give up porn. Ironically enough, it was circumcision that finally penetrated the long-standing emotional fog that I now believe was caused by porn use. Of course, the emotions I was feeling were horrible, but they were at least strong emotions. More than half a year later, I cried for the first time in over a decade. It was in the middle of the night in my bed out of despair and rage from my circumcision. A week later, something else happened that sent me even lower. My best friend in the whole world came to my door and admitted that he'd spent the last 10 minutes sitting in his room holding a knife to his throat, considering killing himself and imagining what it would be like.

"Are you serious?" I asked. He nodded. I looked down at the floor. I looked back up at him. I strongly considered punching him in the face, but instead something ripped deep in my chest and I began to sob. Deep, horrible sobs that washed out everything inside me. I backed away to sit on the edge of my bed, hiding my head in my hands and crying loudly like this for several minutes. I'm crying now thinking about it.

At the time I was thinking that I should do something for him, say something to him, but all I could do was weep. And maybe that was best for the both of us. After I had calmed down, we started talking, and he said that as soon as he saw my reaction he knew he could never commit suicide, as he didn't want to cause his loved ones that pain. I confided that this was the second time I had cried in as little as a week, and then for the first time I told someone what I had learned about circumcision and what I was doing about it. For the record, my friend is whole and had no idea about any of this. Even after I explained it I don't think he really understood, but it was incredibly cathartic to finally tell someone.

At the time porn was definitely a crutch for me. With my failure as a sexual being in real life, sometimes I used porn to reassure myself that I was not just permanently impotent. I would come home from a failed night with a woman and see if I could get an erection with porn. Easy. I thought that proved that I was simply uncomfortable being sexual with another person involved and needed to practice. I did not know at that time what I do now: that repeated porn use creates a separate neurochemical reward pathway in the brain than would be activated by real sex. That by reinforcing this artificial pathway over years, the other is no longer functional. That the only way to heal myself was to rid my life of porn forever and masturbation/fantasy for months (the "reboot") before I could build up the "real sex" pathway (the "rewire"). Here is a snippet from the article "'Sexual Anorexia': Porn May Be Killing Young Men's Sexual Performance":

[…]the Italian study, which surveyed 28,000 pornography users, found that many men may be suffering from 'sexual anorexia.' While it sounds like a bizarrely unbelievable term, the study results seem to corroborate the notion that too much porn has a negative impact on sexual performance. Apparently, men become so accustomed to the unrealistic images they see in pornography that they can no longer get erections.

For many of the men in the Italian study, regular consumption of porn began at age 14, with daily use in their mid-20s including violent images that they had become accustomed to. While gradual, this consumption has apparently harmed their real-life relationships.[30]

I wish this article had existed years ago and I had read it then instead of now.

Since I was unable to explore my sexual preferences in real life, I of course explored them in porn, searching out new and different and generally more extreme categories. I now know that this escalation occurs with every porn addict, and it happens because with such overuse of those pleasure pathways, more extreme and varied content is needed to reach the same level of high (a process called "desensitization"). Much of what I watched increasingly revolved around angry, rough, forceful sex, rape fantasy, and the domination of women. This is also very common, I later learned, because to reach the same high it is easier to combine sexual desire with the cathartic expression of anger. And I certainly had enough anger to go around. I should note that in the case of rape, I only enjoyed fantasizing about rape *fantasy*, in which the woman has stated beforehand that she wants this and may pretend to fight at first but is really loving it. The thought of actual rape—forcing myself on someone who didn't want me—always disgusted me. I have read that some completely heterosexual men even start watching and masturbating to gay porn just because it's a new extreme—a way to get that same level of dopamine in their system that the old stuff just doesn't provide anymore. In the same way, some completely homosexual men begin watching straight or lesbian porn and fetishizing the female genitalia. I have spoken with men who have experienced this and understand how it can happen, but in my case my fixation never strayed from females.

Would I ever have developed my violent sexual desires without porn? Maybe. Unfortunately, every male friend I have watches porn, so I don't have a control group's experiences to draw upon. I have, however, spoken with women who very much enjoy being dominated and role-playing rape fantasy, and at least a couple of these women had no history with or interest in porn. So maybe in a healthy, trusting relationship, it is natural for partners to play with exchanges of power, S&M, and rape fantasy as a positive and cathartic form of sexual

---

[30] Hallowell, B. (2011, October 24). 'Sexual anorexia': Porn may be killing young men's sexual performance. *The Blaze*. Web.

expression. But as part of a porn addiction: no.

I hope that one sentence in particular of that last paragraph raised your eyebrows a bit. I'm talking about the fact that I have no male friends (that I know of) who don't watch porn. I have not spoken with every last one of them about it, but of the dozens I have talked to, every single one watches porn. Men's brains are evolutionarily designed over millions of years to reward sexual congress with a variety of attractive mates, and when several attractive mates are ready and willing, the human male is designed to binge. So what about when hundreds, thousands of mates are easily accessible and waiting right there in your computer? And what if a young male encounters this for the first time when he is 9 or 10 years old with a very malleable and addiction-prone brain? It could be compared to giving a child an unlimited supply of hard drugs, but the truth is that porn is far more naturally addictive to men than alcohol, drugs, or gambling.

I'm sure that like me most of my friends are addicted to porn to some degree and have escalated into categories of porn that at one point they never imagined they'd be turned on by. When I got to college, I was actually relieved to discover the prevalence of porn. I realized that I was no different from any of the other young men there. They all enjoyed Internet porn from a young age. Many had been caught at one time or another, and all had learned to conceal their habit from their families. Looking back, I realize now the connection between this culture of pornography and how many men I had heard say in private that sex was dissatisfying to them and that they had trouble maintaining an erection without oral sex (which, like porn, provides more visual stimulation). Most blamed it on condoms deadening sensation or alcohol, and I'm sure these were factors. After reading the stories of men who have healed from pornography addiction, however, I am fairly certain that porn was the true cause of these men's difficulties. Many also have trouble becoming emotionally involved with their partners or with maintaining interest in a real partner for very long. A serious problem afflicting the majority of my generation of males? The more I think about it, the more it appears that way.

For myself, there were more women, more beds, but I was never able to achieve anything close to a satisfying sexual experience. Though I did tell one of them about my pain and difficulty with circumcision, so I was getting better opening up. In fact, over the last 2 years I have felt like I am in a new puberty—an emotional puberty. The lows seem lower and the highs seem higher. I am more in touch with my own soul than I have ever been. I can be sad and cry. It's like my brain finally said, "Enough is enough," and started to shine through the emotional fog and break down the armor I had built around the image of my masculinity. I even grew enough that I could talk with my family about my circumcision.

After college, my life was fairly bereft of women for a good while. I had had enough sexual failures that I wasn't eager to pursue more, and my sexual confidence was understandably low even as my emotional health was budding. I got jobs, traveled, and had great life experiences. I also watched porn and television and movies a LOT (TV and movies more so than porn, though; my consumption of porn was about the same). Sometimes due to travel or work I would be away from electronics and masturbation for weeks at a time, and thinking that it was probably healthier for me this way, I committed a couple of times to giving up porn. I was still only guessing that porn was a problem for me, however, and without a firm reason to stay away I always slipped back into it.

More recently, I have begun working on more of my art and writing (I have a liberal arts degree). In the past I would work on these artistic projects in bursts, but I would often find it very hard to get motivated and easily slipped into watching TV, playing video games, or masturbating to pornography. But recently, apart from just working on my art, I have been sharing it with people I know and the world at large. Any artist knows that it is a very stressful experience to expose himself/herself in that way. At first I was very concerned with the feedback I was getting and hinged my worth as an artist on whether or not others appreciated my products. As time went on, however, I started caring about this less. I still listened to others' feedback and enjoyed praise, but it no longer bothered me if people didn't like my art or ignored it. I knew that I was doing my best, and I became more secure in my self-worth.

Even more recently, I was at a party. I had gotten to the point at which I can socially do pretty well at parties, but I often had to battle some social anxiety. But on this occasion I found it easy to connect and laugh with anybody there, and I found I could usually control and direct the social situation without too much difficulty, and when I couldn't, I didn't really care and just enjoyed myself. There was a woman there whom I had known from awhile back. I'd always been attracted to her, though I hadn't seen her in years. I was utterly calm and confident in my playful interactions with her, and I knew how to push her buttons from my reading and past experiences. It wasn't appropriate to make a direct move at the time, but when she was leaving we embraced, and she clung tightly against my chest. I put my hands on her hips and held her a few inches from me, looking her directly in the eyes and saying that we needed to see each other soon. She agreed with a grin, and the sexual energy I felt from her was intoxicating.

The simple events of this day came together as the final catalyst in breaking down so much of the weighty, oppressive baggage that I had been carrying around. It was really a culmination of years of progress, but it's like I felt that progress inside of me all at once. I found that over the next couple of days all of my self-doubt, my fear, my embarrassment, my shame, my social anxiety—it was all quickly melting away to be replaced by a feeling of supreme self-assurance. I felt incredible. I feel incredible now. It was like I had been a scared boy all of my life, but now I was a man. In this society it is very difficult for a young male to tell when he becomes a man because we don't have any set coming-of-age ritual, but I didn't need that ritual anymore, because I just *was* a man. I now knew that fact better than I knew my own name. I also knew that I still had possibly my worst demon to face. But while a boy runs or hides from his demons, a man faces them, and I am ready to do that now. I started researching porn addiction and its effects on male sexuality. I guess I knew deep down that porn might be part of my problems. After reading so many stories similar to mine from online communities like this and doing extensive research, I knew I was right. And I found out what I needed to do.

If you are still reading, then at least parts of my story resonate with you. Chances are that you face similar problems. If not, it is extremely likely that some of the men in your life do, and I hope that this text helps you to understand them. Share this book with them so that they may understand themselves.

Dude, you don't watch porn? (prevalence and cultural impact)

From my own experiences I know how much damage consistent porn use can inflict, but how widespread are these problems, really? A recent study of over 800 students (ages 18-26) on six college campuses revealed that 87% of the men and 31% of the women use pornography.[31] To put that 87% into perspective, consider that only 67% of men in the United States use alcohol.[32] (Tellingly, only 67% of men in the study agreed that viewing pornography is acceptable, meaning that quite a few of them use porn despite believing that it is wrong.)

But porn use does not just start at age 18. According to a 2009 University of North Carolina study of young people in the Southeastern United States, over half (53%) of males and nearly a third of females (28%) age 12-15 reported using sexually explicit media. Among the males, this percentage rose drastically from 43.2% of 12-year-olds to 66.1% of 14-year-olds. Among females: from 21.2% at 12 to 38.9% at 14.[33] In Alberta, Canada, a study of 13- and 14-year-olds revealed that one-third of boys were heavy users, having viewed pornographic videos "too many times to count".[34]

So porn use is prevalent. I am not sure which fact is more impressive: that nearly nine out of ten young college men use porn, or that more than one in five 12-year-old girls do. It is more difficult to find hard data that details how all of these people are affected by their porn use, but it seems to do more than threaten sexual and emotional dysfunction. That same UNC study analyzed how the use of sexually explicit material affects adolescents' sexual development. Their

---

[31] Carroll, J., Padilla-Walker, L., Nelson, L., Olson, C., Barry, C., Madsen, S. (2008, January). Generation XXX: Pornography acceptance and use among emerging adults. *Journal of Adolescent Research*, 23, 6-30.

[32] Saad, L. (2012, August 17). Majority in U.S. drink alcohol, averaging four drinks a week. *Gallup Well-Being*. Web.

[33] Brown, J., L'Engle, K. (2009, February). X-Rated: Sexual attitudes and behaviors associated with U.S. early adolescents' exposure to sexually explicit media. *Communication Research*, 36, 129-151.

[34] University of Alberta. (2007, February 25). One In three boys heavy porn users, study shows. *ScienceDaily*. Web.

conclusion: "By the end of middle school many teens have seen sexually explicit content not only on the Internet but in more traditional forms of media as well. Such exposure is related to early adolescents' developing sense of gender roles, sexual relationships, and sexual behavior, including perpetration of sexual harassment."[35]

Yes, porn use has been linked to increased sexual aggressiveness, including sexual harassment and assault. In London the number of sexual offenses committed by children increased 20% from 1,664 cases in 2002/2003 to 1,988 cases in 2006, a jump linked to the greater availability of Internet porn to minors.[36] In Australia in the early 1990's, the Child at Risk Assessment Unit at Canberra Hospital saw about three children under 10 each year who were considered "sexually aggressive". Now, they expect about 70 children each year to fall into this category, "many of whom prey on other children forcing them to take part in sexual acts." Looking for a pattern to explain this trend, social worker Cassandra Tinning examined the case files and found that "almost all those children had accessed the Internet and specifically had accessed the Internet for pornographic material."[37]

This is not to say that any well-adjusted child can be transformed into a sex criminal by Internet porn. Rather, it is children who are predisposed to aggressive behavior due to abuse, neglect, or mental illness who are most suggestible by pornography. Researchers Malamuth, Addison, and Koss found that high-risk individuals who are also heavy porn users are about four times more likely to commit sexually aggressive acts than high-risk males who use porn rarely or never.[38] Those non-users may still act out, but they are much less likely to act out sexually without the influence of pornography.

High-risk adolescents may be the most dramatically affected by porn exposure, but many others experience more subtle effects. In a

---

[35] Brown, J., L'Engle, K. (2009, February). X-Rated: Sexual attitudes and behaviors associated with U.S. early adolescents' exposure to sexually explicit media. *Communication Research*, 36, 129-151.

[36] Web is blamed for 20 per cent leap in sex attacks by children. (2007, March 3). *The Evening Standard*. Web.

[37] Limb, J. (2003, November 26). Alarming rise in children's sexually-abusive behaviour. *The World Today*. Web.

[38] Malamuth, N., Addison, T., Koss, M. (2000). Pornography and sexual aggression: Are there reliable effects and can we understand them? *Annual Review of Sex Research*, 11, 26-91.

review of modern research on exactly these effects, the authors concluded, "research suggests that adolescents who use pornography, especially that found on the Internet, have lower degrees of social integration, increases in conduct problems, higher levels of delinquent behavior, higher incidence of depressive symptoms, and decreased emotional bonding with caregivers" as well as decreased self-confidence.[39]

Even more directly harmful to children—though thankfully on a smaller scale—is child pornography itself, and the number of images on the Internet depicting children in a sexual manner grew fourfold from 2003 to 2007.[40] The extremity of the content has also increased. According to the Internet Watch Foundation in 2008, 58% of the hundreds of assessed domains contain level 4 or 5 material, level 4 being "Penetrative sexual activity involving a child or children, or both children and adults", and level 5 being "Sadism or penetration of or by an animal".[41] Supply follows demand. Over the past decades we have seen the porn supply escalate to more and more extreme content in order to appease an audience that has grown bored with scenes of vanilla sex, which raises the question: Can demand for sexual content involving children be in part driven by heavy porn users who have developed a tolerance and need shocking new genres in order to get off?

Children, of course, grow into adults. Famed psychologist Philip Zimbardo and assistant Nikita Duncan analyze the failing performance (and not just sexually) of the modern man in their book, *The Demise of Guys: Why Boys Are Struggling and What We Can Do About It*. In *Demise*, Zimbardo and Duncan demonstrate that men who grew up during the Internet Age are in general academically failing, socially inept, ADHD-prone layabouts who spend most of their time indulging their "arousal addictions", chiefly featuring pornography and video games but also including social media, television, etc. Men are now 30% more likely than women to drop out of both high school and college. Two-thirds of students in "special education" are males. In private US universities,

---

[39] Owens, E., Behun, R., Manning, J., Reid, R. (2012). The impact of Internet pornography on adolescents: A review of the research. *Sexual Addiction & Compulsivity*, 19, 99-122.

[40] Zheng, Y. (2007, April 16). Watchdog: Online child porn more brutal. *Fox News*. Web.

[41] 2008 annual and charity report. (2008). *IWF Annual Report 2008*. Web.

only 40.7% of students are male.[42] Lastly, boys are more than twice as likely as girls to be diagnosed with attention deficit hyperactivity disorder (ADHD) and thus be treated with brain-altering drugs.[43]

And many suffer from personal and social difficulties that are never diagnosed as a disorder. For instance, 40 years ago, 40% of Americans surveyed agreed that "shyness was a major current trait that they possessed." Today, 60% of Americans say the same, and Zimbardo and Duncan link this change to increased technology use,[44] which minimizes in-person social contact, rendering us bumbling social idiots when we force ourselves to that party or find a date. According to Gary Wilson, the symptoms of arousal addiction—which includes porn addiction—mimic ADHD, social anxiety, depression, performance anxiety, and obsessive-compulsive disorder.[45] The diagnosis rate for many of these disorders has risen sharply in recent years.

Concerning sexual performance, doctors are seeing more and more young men complaining of sexual difficulty. Erectile dysfunction was once the realm of older men with 60 years of bacon grease under their belts (and lining their arteries), but now one patient in four diagnosed with ED is a young man,[46] and that just accounts for those smart enough to go to a doctor. Because of embarrassment or other factors, many more men than that are fueling a thriving black market of non-prescription ED drugs.[47] Thousands of websites sell ED drugs or

---

[42] Borzelleca, D. (2012, February 16). The male-female ratio in college. *Forbes*. Web.

[43] Bloom, B., Jones, L., Freeman, G. (2013, December). Summary health statistics for
U.S. children: National Health Interview Survey, 2012. National Center for Health Statistics. *Vital and Health Statistics*, 10 (258).

[44] Zimbardo, P. G., & Duncan, N. (2012). *The demise of guys why boys are struggling and what we can do about it*. New York: Ted Conferences.

[45] TEDx Talks. (2012, May 16). The great porn experiment: Gary Wilson at TEDxGlasgow. *YouTube*. Web.

[46] Capogrosso, P., Colicchia, M., Ventimiglia, E., Castagna, G., Clementi, M. C., Suardi, N., Castiglione, F., Briganti, A., Cantiello, F., Damiano, R., Montorsi, F. and Salonia, A. (2013). One patient out of four with newly diagnosed erectile dysfunction is a young man—worrisome picture from the everyday clinical practice. *Journal of Sexual Medicine*, 10, 1833–1841.

[47] Carey, T. (2012, October 3). Addicted to Viagra: They should be at their most virile, but a growing number of young men can't cope without those little blue pills. *Mail Online*. Web.

"herbal remedies" at reduced prices, peddling over two million pills each month. Even if men were getting exactly what they thought they were buying, consistent use of ED drugs can be harmful to one's health, but many of these pills sold online are counterfeit or inadequately labeled, containing potentially dangerous active ingredients or no active ingredients at all.[48]

Porn-using men and women, of course, still get married. Just over two million marriages are performed every year in the United States; during that same time, more than a million marriages end in divorce. At the November 2002 meeting of the American Academy of Matrimonial Lawyers, 350 attorneys were surveyed to determine if the Internet played a significant role in the divorces they handled. 62% said yes, and of these, "56 percent of the divorce cases involved one party having an obsessive interest in pornographic websites."[49]

It is not hard to see how porn addiction may harm marriage. In 1988—before widespread home Internet connectivity—researchers Dolf Zillman and Jennings Bryant sought to understand how regular pornography use affects happiness. Participants were shown either pornographic (of the non-violent, vanilla variety) or non-pornographic videos in several sessions over six weeks. After this time, participants rated their happiness and satisfaction concerning various facets of their lives. Results show that this exposure to pornography had no appreciable effects on any aspect of their happiness except one: their satisfaction with their sexual lives and relationships. Specifically, participants reported decreased satisfaction with their "partners' affection, physical appearance, sexual curiosity, and sexual performance [...] In addition, subjects assigned increased importance to sex without emotional involvement. These effects were uniform across gender."[50]

If just one hour viewing pornography per week over six weeks can result in significant dissatisfaction with one's partner, imagine how badly an Internet porn addict's relationship may suffer when he comes to prefer cumpilation videos to his wife's embrace, sabotages trust by lying about his habit, develops porn-induced sexual dysfunction, begins to use her as an aid to masturbation while fantasizing about more

---

[48] Buying ED drugs online: What's the risk?. *WebMD*. Web.

[49] Manning, J. (2005, August). The impact of Internet pornography on marriage and the family: A review of the research. Web.

[50] Zillmann, D. and Bryant, J. (1988). Pornography's impact on sexual satisfaction. *Journal of Applied Social Psychology*, 18, 438–453.

stimulating porn-like scenes, or escalates to using prostitutes or online/offline affairs. One wife of a heavy porn user gives us a typical yet poignant example of a marriage threatened by porn addiction.

Pwidow: *Hello, I am 34, I have been married for nearly 8 years and for the second (serious, outside of dropping hints) time confronted my husband about what I believed to be a very serious porn addiction. The first time I confronted him about it was after he came back from Iraq and we didn't have sex for nearly a week after he returned. During that time, I found him downloading a "bittorrent" of a particular porn star that I found out later "was a favorite." When I looked at his search history, I found that he had been looking porn stars up by name as well, which devastated me. I had just had two babies inside two years, and there was no way I could compete with these women with perfect bodies. I felt so heartbroken, and it felt like cheating and I said so. My husband responded that this was how he coped with his "needs" *without* cheating. So fast forward almost 4 years and our sex life was a shadow of what it used to be. Once a month maybe, and he was noticeably softer and sometimes couldn't finish. I caught him in our garage room office PM'ing in the middle of the day when he was supposed to be working on the house. He would sneak looks while playing computer games, when I wasn't around. He disengaged. It was almost as if he was a sociopath: he didn't seem to care when I would cry about our love life, his porn use, his lack of interest in our family. He would tell me he loved me and the kids, but it seemed so mechanical.*

During these years, I stopped taking care of myself. I have always been told I am attractive, but I let myself get fat, I would shower once or twice a week. I was a great mom, feeding my kids organic, but I didn't do ANY exercise, and I ate whatever without any regard to calories. I got lost in Facebook as a means to adult interaction (as we were military and would move to places where I had no friends), which ended up becoming MY addiction. I just fell into this abyss of self-hate because I wasn't good enough. He even joked to a friend that "why should he do dishes to get a BJ if he could just look at porn."

While this may sound awful, I had dated much better looking and "with-it" guys prior to my husband, and what attracted me to him—and led me to marry him—was that he was a GOOD GUY. He seemed like the perfect family man and someone that would treat me like a queen forever. Of course I was also attracted to him, but his looks and social standing were not quite on par with previous. Then again those previous with a higher social standing and better looks also ended up being assholes. I digress.

What brought all of this to a head was a recent one-year overseas tour (he is still currently on for less than 5 months). Right before he left, we had not had sex in at least a month, maybe two. I said the night before he left that I really wanted to have sex since I would not see him again for a while and so we did. He had a hard time maintaining an erection and he could not orgasm that night. I felt like a failure. I felt like I was ugly and unwanted. I cried and he said it was because he thought I wasn't enjoying myself and that I was only doing it because he was leaving. Before this, our marriage, well, sucked. I had a lot of pent up resentment from him not wanting to do any outside family activities (I took the kids to the pumpkin patch by myself because he didn't like doing "that stuff"). He would bitch when I wanted to take the kids to the fair. He allowed our daughter to get out of the house in nothing but a diaper, while he was "on the toilet" as I was gone for 45 minutes dropping our son off, having the police come knocking on our door asking if that was our daughter as I pull up. It all makes sense now, as I read about hypofrontality and the antisocial behavior that develops with increased porn use. I wasn't crazy! He HAD changed.

So I made a pact to myself that while he was gone, I would better myself. And I did. So far I have lost 35 pounds and went from a size 18/20 to a 12/14. I have stopped using Facebook as a crutch and started living life more. Though the latter more recently. I have engaged with my kids more, started hanging out with friends more, even though I would've liked nothing more than to remain a hermit. I look GREAT now, I shower daily. I have gone out and have had 21-year-old boys hit on me. Things were going well, it seemed. Little did I know, the worst was yet to come. I thought that by bettering myself, my husband would love me more and want me more.

I caught him this summer chatting inappropriately with a former lover online, I don't think it went too far, but it went far enough that I felt betrayed. We made up, after talking, where he railed at me and told me that I was just feeling guilty for being a bad wife and that's why I snooped on him. He finally apologized, though not sincerely enough for me, and agreed to work on us.

He came home for leave a few months later and, considering our trust issues, I snooped the hell out of his phone. He had it mostly wiped clean, but I did find an app that he had uninstalled for "sweet discreet" and I made a fake profile and found his on there. It was clearly a picture of himself and an entire profile created on what he was looking for, which was very porny sex—no strings attached. I confronted him and after repeated denials, he finally admitted he did it while drunk and upset one night, but he couldn't remember the fake email and password to delete it, and he had never physically cheated on me (Which he still hasn't done to this day—delete it). During this time he was home my drive was through the roof (exercise!), and while we did have sex many times, it always seemed like he had to slam it in to keep it hard, and he was handling himself a couple times between positions, and a couple times he couldn't O—and the last few days, he just wasn't in the mood and complained of being tired.

I also was able to find the email address he had attached to his new phone and after he left, I logged into it about a week after he had returned overseas. In his account portion, I was able to see what he had searched and I nearly died. Not only was he having 8 hour porn binges (like the one he had the day he got back after seeing us (a day after he was "too tired"), but the CONTENT was SO disturbing. Just utter debasement of women with just awful things. I won't go into detail, but needless to say it was beyond kinky and just outright deviant and perverted—luckily only involving grown women. And he was actively searching these things out and watching them for hours. So, after searching online I found YBOP and as terrible as this sounds, I felt so much better. I remember when I had found his search history before, it had never included things like these. I confronted him about the more "benign" things I found, and he became incensed. I had violated his privacy (which I had, but as his wife with trust issues, I felt somewhat vindicated), I was "embarrassing him on purpose", he "just couldn't talk to me" and he didn't for almost 2 days. I finally wrote him a lengthy email where I told him about what I had watched (the 6 part series on YBOP), that it fit him, and that I knew what he was searching, all of it, and his year-ago self would be horrified. He finally agreed that he has a problem and said he would "try" to give it up cold turkey. He has watched 4 of the 6 part series, and I even linked the page for support groups for him. He seems really on board, but part of me can't help but wonder if he is giving me lip service, if his heart is really in it, or if he can do it on his own without me to help him be accountable.

To be clear, I was a really crappy wife for the past few years. I had given up just as much as him, I suppose, in my own way. But, I am feeling alive and great and I just want my husband back. I want to be a happy, engaged, fully living family. I also want the really great sex that my husband and I had, and still can have back!

In Schneider's survey of partners of cybersex addicts, she found that the addiction had created severe problems of mistrust, resentment, sexual dissatisfaction, separation, neglect and harm to any children, and divorce. Among 68% of the couples, one or both partners had lost interest in sex with the other. Partners reported loss of self-esteem, hopelessness about being able to compete with online women, and pain in reaction to online affairs as severe as they would feel in reaction to offline affairs. 37.1% of respondents with children reported that "The kids have lost parental time and attention/lost their 2-parent home." 30% reported that "The children have seen us argue, see the stress in the home [related to cybersex addiction]." 14.3% reported that "The children have seen pornography and/or masturbation and I'm worried for them." 11.4% reported that "The children have seen the pornography and have been adversely affected."[51]

Brothers, we are not doing so well. Too many of us have slipped from casual to compulsive porn/cybersex use, and our individual struggles are manifesting on a cultural, global level. It is not our fault that we live in an environment filled with unnaturally powerful temptations, but it is our duty to ourselves, our families, and our communities to be the best men that we can be. In order to become our best, we must recognize when our temptations start to become problems—then we must find solutions.

---

[51] Schneider, J. (2000). Effects of cybersex addiction on the family: Results of a survey. *jenniferschneider.com*. Web.

Part Two: The Solution

I feel like toasted **** (what to expect when you quit)

If you are a compulsive porn user, then before deciding whether or not to quit you need to know what to expect out of the journey that is a porn-free life. Men who have made this journey before you have encountered the following before considering themselves healed and free of addiction. You will likely live several of these experiences but are unlikely to encounter all of them.

Time. The amount of weeks or months that it takes to heal yourself of problem symptoms will depend on many factors. Most notably, older men who did not start masturbating to Internet porn until they were adults seem to have an easier time returning to healthy sexual function than do younger men who started PMO during their formative adolescent or teenage years. Presumably this is because users who began using earlier in their lives—when their brains were most highly adaptive and malleable—conditioned themselves more thoroughly for porn, especially if porn use came before any real sexual experiences.

The length of the journey also depends on the severity of your symptoms, how often and how you masturbate during the process, relapses to PMO, the opportunity to rewire with real partners, and your emotional state. Most men continue to see improvement even in the months and years after they consider themselves healed and are enjoying a healthy sex life—whatever that may be for them. Mild addicts and older men may hope for good results in as little as a few weeks, while younger long-term users often see good improvement after several months. Even fully committed, however, it may take some men close to a year to heal. No one who has committed to the process, however, has failed to see results, even if they came later than was expected or preferred.

Hypersexuality and cravings. As an addict, your body and brain are very likely used to consistent sexual outlet. When they stop watching porn and masturbating, many men quickly feel a sharp increase in sex drive that usually lasts for a few days to a week or more. They may experience spontaneous erections throughout the day. Many will fail at this first obstacle, perhaps thinking that this short time away from porn was all they needed, and it will not hurt to masturbate just once or twice. In fact, their body *needs* the release, they rationalize. But this is not yet a return of the natural sexual impulse. These urges are not a need of the body for release but actually the dopamine cravings of an addicted brain crying out for a fix. One man recalls a recent craving.

Jeff: *That was probably the biggest urge I have ever had in my life. It was just so incredibly intense. I was honestly not in a place to have any rational thought, but somehow I noticed the tiny part of my rational mind that told me to take two minutes out to cool down so and closed my laptop and sat down and meditated in front of my little Buddha shrine in my room. I only managed about 5 minutes because I was in such a dopamine frenzy but it was enough to make me calm enough to stop me relapsing. [...] It was a* very *close shave.*

Flatline. Near total lack of sexual drive and erections, often accompanied by depression and apathy. Sometimes called "dead dick", most men encounter flatline at least once while in recovery. Usually it occurs after the hypersexuality phase, though many enter a flatline right after quitting PMO and some may not experience flatline until several months into their journeys. A man can alternate between flatline and hypersexuality as his body and brain go through the changes necessary for a return to natural sexual and emotional function. In flatline, many men begin to fear that this is it. This is their new life, and they'll never recover their sexual fire. In desperation they use porn to tease out a sexual response and end up relapsing. But flatline is a strong sign that real changes are occurring in the limbic system, and it will end.

Anonymous: *Unlike a lot of people here, during the first few days I didn't get extremely horny, etc. Instead for my first 45 days I basically flatlined and had dead dick. No erections, no urge for sex, no libido. Nothing. It was extremely scary as I really thought something was medically wrong with me. During the first half I also experienced depression on some days that was pretty severe.*

Emotional turmoil. As the neurochemical receptors in porn addicts' brains begin to re-sensitize, many men experience a wide range of powerful emotions. These emotions can manifest in almost any way imaginable, from sublime wonder at the beauty of nature to despair-induced panic attacks, from blinding rage at the empty juice carton left in the fridge to sobbing at baby powder commercials in between football quarters. But as addicts' bodies find a new balance, these emotional outbursts do normalize.

Anonymous: *Excessive porn viewing and masturbation dampened my ability to feel emotions to their fullest. I had my first good cry in several years after about ten days into one of my early streaks. Since then, I've cried many times—*

while listening to music, reading a story, thinking about people in my life, even beautiful ideas can make me emotional. This wasn't the case before. For as long as I can remember, I had been melancholy and generally unaffected by the world around me. Certain things were powerful enough to cut through the haze I lived in, but mostly I floated. I was uncomfortably numb. The reversal of this has been one of the more profound changes I've seen since quitting, and has been particularly rewarding. Emotional sensitivity has given rise to increasingly frequent bursts of creativity. Being moved by something you've created is truly rewarding, and incredibly reinforcing. I've written more music that I'm actually proud of in the last few months than I have in the previous four years.

Vivid, dark dreams. It is very common to begin dreaming more clearly while healing, and often dreams become more disturbingly sexual, at least in the beginning. Men commonly dream at least once about relapsing to porn, usually struggling against it even while giving in. As their journeys progress, these visions usually give way to a higher frequency of dreams about desirable sex.

Nocturnal emissions. Occurrence of "nocturnal emissions" or "wet dreams" can increase when abstaining from other sexual activity. The dreamer usually experiences a sexual dream and wakes up to find he is ejaculating or has already ejaculated. Even those who have never had a nocturnal emission in their lives may begin to experience them during this journey. Emissions are not considered to be a setback or relapse, though some men experience a reduction in libido and energy after these events. Accidental ejaculation can happen during waking hours as well, and though this is rare it is no more of a relapse unless brought about with fantasy or purposeful physical stimulation.

A new life (how to heal—permanently)

Some people are able to use porn in moderation and seemingly still enjoy fulfilling emotional and sexual relationships. If you self-qualify as an addict based on the criteria I gave earlier and/or are experiencing undesirable symptoms from your porn use and masturbation, then you are not one of these people.

You have already read about how PMO can alter us and what benefits we may see upon quitting, but what comes in between is our transformation. I do not use that word lightly. Quitting PMO is not a cure-all that will change us into our ideal selves, but it does help clear the way for greater changes, which in turn will give us strength and reason not to return to bad old habits. This journey is not about altering just one aspect of our lives: it is about transforming ourselves into men who no longer require such artificial, empty satisfaction. Some will find it not very difficult to stop using porn, and by now those of you in this group have the information you need to decide if this is what you want to do. Many who want to quit, however, find themselves facing severe cravings and relapsing several times before realizing that they may not have the ability to break through this addiction without help. This guide is specifically for those men, but anyone who wants to leave behind his vices and strengthen himself and his relationships may benefit from it.

There are only two real paths available to the problematic porn user.

Path #1: This one is easy. Continue to enjoy porn. After all, it feels good, right? PMO is a great way to handle stress, pass the time, explore your sexuality, deal with (read: avoid) emotional problems, and just relax. And everyone does it, so it can't be that bad.

Path #2: Realize how much porn use has hurt you and that PMO is completely incompatible with the person you want to be. Immediately delete/throw away/burn every bit of your porn collection and commit to healing yourself, no matter what temptations you face, depressions you sink into, or rationalizations your addiction whispers into your ear. Face the good and the bad of the coming months with equal determination, and emerge on the other side a stronger, happier, more fulfilled man enjoying all of the benefits of his natural sexuality.

These are your choices, and the hard fact is that many of you are not ready for path #2. Perhaps you have not yet sunk low enough to be motivated along that path. Wait until you start being unable to reach orgasm or maintain an erection with a partner. Wait until you realize that you are unable to form an emotional connection with a woman or think of her as more than a toy. Wait until you escalate the content of the porn you watch to a point at which you disgust yourself or begin to doubt your own natural hetero- or homosexuality. Perhaps then you will be desperate enough to commit to path #2. When that time comes, pick up this book again. For now, go cruise PornHub.

Most porn addicts who encounter all of this information, whether it be through a TED talk, a friend, or this book, will try to walk down path #3.

Path #3: PMO has hurt you, sure, and yes you need to take a break for awhile and greatly reduce your use, but *never* watch porn again? Don't talk crazy! You can enjoy all the benefits of quitting porn while still occasionally indulging. At least save a few of your favorite videos to your hard drive just for old times' sake.

Path #3 sounds pretty good, right? Unfortunately, there are major drawbacks to keeping porn as a part of your life—even a very small part. Path #2 leads to freedom. You may face strong cravings for several weeks or several months, but over time the PMO pathways in your brain will wither away and your sexual energy will refocus toward real-life partners. PMO will be a thing of your past, and you will no longer have to fight cravings for it. On path #3, porn always remains a possibility, and so those pathways will never die; you will fight your cravings constantly. One PMO will turn into two will turn into a binge, and you will feel shame and guilt for not having the willpower to moderate yourself.

You do not need to give a dog a treat every time it does a trick in order for it to continue following commands; you only need to give it a treat occasionally. It is the *possibility* of a treat that keeps the dog a slave to old habits. If you withhold treats for long enough, eventually the dog will stop obeying your commands, and if you abstain from PMO for long enough, eventually you will lose interest in it and move on with your life. Ultimately, path #3 is not a path at all, and those who try to follow it are merely hacking their way zigzag through the jungle just to find themselves back on path #1. They enjoy the smooth, well-trod path #1 for awhile, then square their shoulders and march back into the jungle to find path #3, catching themselves on vines and tripping over roots before again stumbling back to PMO.

Forgive the metaphor, but you understand my point. I have seen many "senior members" of online support groups for porn and masturbation addicts with hundreds or thousands of posts over months and years to their names but with "PMO Trackers" that read, "2 days, 7 hours since I last PMO'd" or "4 days, 11 hours since I last looked at P." These men know the facts, and they see themselves as being in a constant struggle with their PMO addictions that will one day culminate in them being healed. Unfortunately, many of these men are losing that struggle because they are not ready to commit. They are not truly ready leave PMO behind.

Path #2 seems hard—and it is—but if you are ready for it then I and many other successful men can help guide you with the following steps.

1. Get angry. If you have read this far and consider yourself a porn addict, then your habit has insidiously impacted every part of your life. You have been wasting your best years chasing an empty dopamine high when you could have been building valuable relationships, accomplishing personal goals, and contributing to your community and to the world. Cultivate a disgust for the waste that is PMO. Righteous anger is good motivation to take charge of your life and heal yourself, and it will help tide you through the dark times when you are tempted to return to your habit. But anger and disgust can only take you so far. No one can or should be angry all the time; this would be very unhealthy and ultimately lead to depression, despair, and a return to PMO. See step two.

2. Get excited. By now you have read about all of the benefits that you will enjoy by getting past your porn addiction. You will have more energy, confidence, focus, and sexual strength than you ever remember experiencing. You will leave behind shame, self-doubt, secrets and lies. Do you not want to reach this state as quickly as possible? Anger and disgust at your addiction and your past self will help you start this journey, but in order to remain strong and committed over long days and weeks, focus on your hope for the future. Each day you resist temptation is one day closer to the better tomorrow that you want and that is within your grasp.

3. Get informed. Knowledge is power, and you need to know everything that you can learn about porn addiction and recovery. This book is a solid foundation, but it is up to you to seek out the scientific and anecdotal information that best relates to your journey. Upon entering a flatline, many men fear that they will never recover or feel sexual pleasure again, so out of desperation they test themselves with porn and end up relapsing. If they knew that almost every recovering man enters flatline and that it is one of the strongest signs of real progress, then they would be more likely to hold onto hope and push through hard times.

Often people feel as though they are the only ones to experience their problems. Female porn addicts are especially vulnerable to this false belief as porn is often considered a predominantly male interest, but this is an illusion. There are billions of humans on this planet, and there are no unique problems. Thanks to the Internet, it is no longer difficult to dispel the illusion of being alone with your issues, but you have to pursue the information. To help you do this, there are many valuable tools in the "Additional resources" section at the end of this text. Take advantage. Read both general information and individual stories. If you still have questions, post them to one of the many online communities built around recovery.

4. Purge. You have a sexual history, even if you are a never-been-kissed virgin. Write it down in all of its brutal specificity, no matter how grisly, embarrassing, or pathetic parts of it may be. You need not describe each romantic encounter in erotic detail, but if you leave something out because it shames you then you are cheating yourself out of the benefits of this step. The writing process will serve as an introspective journey into your past, and when you finish you will have a better understanding of your own story and how you became the man that you need to change. As I said above, knowledge is power, and this step will teach you what no other source can: self-knowledge. End this project by writing down your mission and your goals: what you want to accomplish and what benefits you hope to earn. One of those goals may be to confront and come to terms with parts of your past (such as sexual abuse or other trauma) that play a role in your current addiction.

Whatever your goals, when writing them it is important to compose them in a way that facilitates their success. Enter the **SMART** acronym. A goal should be **S**pecific, **M**easurable, **A**chievable, **R**ealistic, and **T**ime-bound. Your goal may be to leave behind PMO forever. Good. Now be specific as to why this is important to you, how you are going to make this happen, and how you will measure progress. And include a plan for dealing with relapse.

Example: *I am 27 years old and my dick doesn't work half the time, no matter how attracted I am to my partner. After researching my problem online, I realized that my ED is probably caused by my heavy porn use over the last several* *years. Now that I realize how much I've hurt myself with porn, I:*

• *commit to never use porn again, nor to masturbate to any artificial media.*

• *will not masturbate or fantasize at all for 90 days, after which I will decide if I want to reintroduce it into my life.*

• *will not have an orgasm for at least 30 days, after which I will decide if I am ready to start reaching orgasm with my partner again or if my sexual response system needs time to recover my erection strength.*

• *will track my progress with a journal, and if I violate any of these goals then I will record how it happened, plan for how to not let it happen again, and resume my mission. I will not let a relapse mean failure, nor will I allow it to be an excuse to binge.*

• *will share everything with my significant other this weekend. I have kept my past and my addiction to myself for too long, and I realize I need help to move forward. If we feel like it's necessary, we'll find a therapist as well.*

Look back at your goals frequently, and when you feel that you have outgrown them or they are not working for you, make your **SMART** goals **SMARTER** by **E**valuating and **R**evising them.

5. Burn bridges. You have a porn collection. It might be DVDs under your mattress, magazines in your sock drawer, bookmarked streaming videos, saved files on your hard drive—whatever. Delete it. Burn it. Throw it all away. This step is absolutely essential. If you save even one favorite video or picture "just in case" then you doom your journey from the starting line because you accept defeat, accept that porn is still a part of your life.

6. Abstain and reboot. The first leg of the healing process is known as the "reboot". Its purpose is to give your sexual response system a rest and allow your neurological dependency on PMO to weaken so that you can replace it with a stronger desire for real partners. But because this wiring for PMO is so strong and easily reinforced, it is imperative that you avoid all sexual stimulation that is not a real, attractive person in front of you. Avoid not just porn but any sexy image, online interface, fantasy, etc. Do not creep on sexy Facebook photos. Do not cruise Craigslist personals. Do not read erotic accounts. Do not watch television or movies with triggering material. Do not linger on that photo of an attractive woman in the newspaper. Do not fantasize. Do not masturbate.

This is where advice diverges depending on whom you ask and what case you consider. Some believe that fantasy and masturbation is fine and even beneficial as long as the fantasy is far removed from porn-like scenes. These men will tell you to focus on using your imagination to create a narrative involving real people in your life. Use a first-person perspective and imagine the progression of intimacy, the smell, the touch of skin against skin. Avoid skipping right to the hardcore scenes, visualizing things you have seen in porn, or using a third-person perspective. These men believe that this type of fantasy helps to rewire your brain to more realistic sexual expectations.

Another option is—if you are able—to masturbate only to sensation. Imagine nothing, look at nothing provocative. Look at the door or your penis, and enjoy only the physical sensations. Many men use this as a test to see if their reboot was successful, as they once needed intense visual or mental stimulation to maintain erection and reach orgasm.

How well either of these options work or whether they are the right approaches for you depends entirely on your individual situation. The distinct disadvantage of these methods is that they do not allow your sexual response system the rest that many recovering addicts find necessary. For men who cannot find a partner to rewire with, these may be good recourses after an initial reboot of complete abstention; they are certainly better than relapsing to porn.

However, masturbation to fantasy or sensation is still masturbation, and more natural masturbation is probably not your end goal. If you want healthy, enjoyable sex with a partner and are having trouble achieving it, then masturbation of any type will likely slow your progress. This is especially true for men who have noticed physical desensitization of the penis due to consistent masturbation. The best way to re-sensitize the penis to the touch of a partner is with complete abstention. The same applies to fantasy without masturbation. The more you do it, the more you reinforce the habit that sexual arousal happens when you are alone and in your head rather than with a partner and focused on real stimuli.

Around this time is when men realize how powerful their addictions are and whether they are more dependent on porn or if the porn habit is built on top of a more deeply rooted need for fantasy. You have to decide for yourself if life would be better in the long term with or without sexual fantasy and masturbation, but abstaining at least during your reboot will likely quicken the healing process.

Additionally, in terms of getting over your addiction "edging" is no better and perhaps worse than MO. Edging is masturbation without orgasm and usually involves approaching climax and then pulling back several times, resulting in longer sessions. People enjoy doing this because they are addicted to the dopamine rush that porn or fantasy provide. These users think that indulging does them no harm as long as they avoid ejaculation, but they are wrong. You do not need to orgasm in order to reinforce your PMO or MO addiction, and edging is relapsing. In terms of dopamine re-sensitization, edging is more harmful than PMO because by delaying orgasm we lengthen the heightened dopamine exposure.

Beware "testing" yourself. There will be many moments along your journey when you wonder whether or not you are making progress. Are you healed yet? How will you know when it happens? You probably want to be sure that you are over whatever problems you have faced before pursuing new partners or reopening sex with your current partner, so you figure you have to test yourself. This mentality can easily lead to relapse, so do not test too soon before your commitment has been cemented by action. If you do decide to test, make sure that you come to this decision over several days of reasoned thinking—not in the heat of the moment or on a whim. Many men agree that after a 60- or 90-day reboot is the best time to test. They recommend using only sensation—no fantasy or visualization. Again, decide well beforehand whether you want only to try to achieve an erection or also to masturbate to orgasm.

Not testing yourself *by* yourself is also an option. How you perform alone is probably not a good predictor of how you will respond to a partner; many men who undertake this journey realize that their natural sex drive is dormant until actually needed. They are not distracted throughout each day with spontaneous erections or a mental preoccupation with sex, but when the moment comes with a real partner, their bodies respond.

Going without sexual release for weeks (much less months) may seem daunting, especially if you have come to rely on masturbation to suppress emotions, to fall asleep, or for any other reason. Sometimes it will feel as if your craving for porn or masturbation will just keep growing and growing until you have to give in, but this is an illusion. Craving comes in waves, and all you need to do to reach still waters again is to remain focused and let the wave pass. There is no physiological requirement to masturbate or orgasm.

7. Avoid triggers. "Triggers" are cues or influences that start you back down the path to PMO. Triggers may be obvious, such as sexual pop-up advertisements, Facebook photos, or television scenes. They may also be more subtle, such as being alone in your room with a laptop, performing an activity that you usually follow with PMO, or texting with a crush. It is especially important during the first few weeks of a reboot that you shun triggers as much as possible, though once you have built a solid foundation of strength and abstention you should find it easier to ignore triggers that only weeks ago would have sent you to your room with a box of tissues.

You must do some critical thinking about what your triggers may be in order to preempt them. Be honest with yourself. If you usually masturbate in the shower, start taking cold showers instead. If you use your phone to view porn, then install filtering software or downgrade to a phone without Internet connectivity. If you usually PMO with your laptop in your room, maybe you only use your computer in the common room of your house now. If you live alone, maybe you only use it in the coffee shop down the street. In that case, maybe you do not even need Internet access in your home anymore, and you can avoid triggers and save money at the same time. If cruising an online dating site or app gets you horny, then it is time to delete your account. If you subscribe to magazines that tempt you, cancel your subscriptions. If you watch TV regularly that includes sexy scenes, then relax by reading the newspaper or exercising instead. Or if you have realized that TV is a drain on your life altogether, maybe it is time to take a sledgehammer to it in the backyard. A memorable and dramatic action like this can serve to cement your commitment to change (and it'll be fun).

Many men use web protection software like K9 to block adult content from their devices. Software like this can be helpful, but it is not flawless. Do not substitute it for your own willpower. Its best function is to prevent accidental viewings and give you a little more time to change your mind as you are desperately trying to deactivate it in a dopamine craze. I also recommend ad-prevention software to block potential triggers, such as Adblock Plus for Firefox. See "Additional resources" for more information on these tools.

Substances are a common trigger. If you get horny and lose willpower after using alcohol, marijuana, etc., then reduce your use or cut those substances out of your life completely—at least for the duration of your reboot.

If in doubt as to whether something is a trigger, there is a simple test you can perform. Are you turned on or experiencing an increased urge to MO due to some stimulus or situation that is not a real partner? Yes? Then stop immediately and preempt that trigger so that it does not threaten your progress again.

8. Track. Monitor your progress, both subjectively and objectively. Subjectively, keep a journal in which you write your feelings, goals, experiences, temptations, etc. Be sure to take note of when you are victorious over temptation and what helps you do so. Objectively, mark days on a calendar or otherwise. If you are successfully abstaining, then each day marked off should add pride to your accomplishment and put another brick into the wall between your new life and your old one.

If you relapse, though, then a counter can serve as a reminder of your failure and an excuse to binge after one reset. In this case merely tracking the length of a streak starts to do more harm than good, and you should instead or in addition keep a spreadsheet that counts each relapse, the nature of the relapse, and the stimuli you relapsed to. Add whatever other details you think will be useful to you. This spreadsheet method helps reinforce the fact that progress is not always all-or-nothing and that relapse is a setback but not a complete reset to your former self. After all, going from PMO every day or several times per week to just once or twice in a month is a huge step in the right direction.

9. Share. Yes, this journey is about to get difficult. **Purge** taught you about your own emotional damage, and now is the time to truly start repairing it. To do so you must share your past history and present struggle with others. The easy way to start opening up is by posting to an anonymous online support community. I posted my story and kept a journal on the forum "Your Brain Rebalanced", but there are several options. These communities can be a great source of information and emotional support, but do not stop at sharing anonymously. You need at least one person in your real life to whom you can open up. There are two reasons for this. First, the people you tell in real life can provide more concrete support for you on your journey (though they may not).

Second, and most importantly, you must break through the barriers that you have set up over the years to keep your ego safe. You do not need them anymore. Not only do these barriers keep other people out: they also keep you locked in. Do you really want to live your whole life subject to shame, never being able to fully and proudly disclose yourself to your friends and family? Everyone has secrets, weaknesses, and problems. Most people will not see you as weak for being an addict but will admire your strength in admitting it, and they will help you through your journey. But even if they spurn you, it does not matter because this journey is for you—not for them. Most users keep secret how deeply they have delved into porn and how it has affected their lives, and they do this out of fear: fear of judgment, embarrassment, shame. But fear only has power over us until we confront its source. When the unknown becomes known, fear melts away. Many addicts of all types use because they doubt their own value and the worth of the lives they lead; indulging in addictions can temporarily distract them from this pain. The true power of this step is that by sharing yourself you accept yourself, and by accepting yourself you acknowledge your own value—acquiring a sense of self-worth that can be an ever-present source of strength. This is your life, and it is time to stop hiding.

Since you have already written your story down, you are now much more able to articulate it to others. You do not need to tell them everything right away, but tell them that you are struggling with what you recently realized is a porn addiction that has negatively impacted your life. If they accept this and are interested in knowing more and helping you, inform them about rebooting and rewiring and how you hope it will help your individual issues. Consider sharing your written story. Who knows, discussing your issues might inspire others to confront their own problematic porn use.

If you have a romantic partner, it is extremely important to share this journey with him or her. In all likelihood he/she will be relieved that you have opened up and be willing to help you through this process (and our partners are the ones best able to help us, so it is essential to have them fully informed and on our team). If you try to keep your partner in the dark in order to maintain your dignity, you will only put that much more pressure on yourself to perform (if you have PIED, DE, or PE), which will make it more difficult to perform. Your partner will know that there is something wrong and may or may not have the courage to ask about it. Either way, if you fail to discuss your problems then the unspoken becomes oppressive and is liable to corrupt and end the relationship. Many, many relationships have withered and died because of porn addiction, and most are due to the addict's inability to talk about his problems or his unwillingness to face them. Do not make the same mistake that so many of us have regretted.

Gerry Blasingame is a counselor who treats sexually compulsive developmentally disabled persons. In treating these people, Blasingame mapped the path to destructive sexual action in the form of a ladder.[52] The top rung is "Bad Sex Behavior", but to get there one has to climb the lower steps. The first rung on the ladder: "Feel Bad". As recovering addicts of any kind know, it is not when we are filled with hope and motivation that we are vulnerable to a relapse. Instead, we are tempted in the hard moments when we are depressed, distraught, or tired. Feeling bad is an unavoidable part of life, so you will find yourself on the first rung of the ladder to relapse often.

The second rung is "Keep It to Myself." Addiction thrives on isolation and secrecy. When we keep our pain private, it can seem overwhelming and insurmountable and lead us back to dark places. But the mere act of sharing your struggle with another person can lighten the burden immensely—like turning on the lights in a dark room to realize that the imagined burglar is really your kitten, Sparkles. Whether it be with a friend, family member, counselor, religious leader, or romantic partner, share your journey with at least one person. Make yourself vulnerable and request help if you need it. Ask for permission to call and talk when you are facing temptation and need a friend. Not only will you improve your chances for success, but you will forge deeper, stronger relationships with your loved ones. We cannot avoid stepping onto the first rung, but often all it takes to get back onto solid ground is the help of a friend.

If you do not trust yourself to succeed alone and need a friend to help you not use, consider installing "accountability software" onto your devices. Such software monitors your online activity and sends reports to an email address of your choosing. See the "Additional resources" section.

10. Fill the void. Quitting PMO does not fix your problems, but it does open the door, allowing you to step forward and take actions that will truly change your life for the better and forever. Once you begin to abstain, you may realize that you used PMO in order to regulate emotions, cover up negative feelings, and/or avoid having to confront your greater responsibilities and goals. It will not work just to remove PMO and hope for the best. You must fill the empty space left in your life by your absent addiction. Try not to resort too much to alternative escapism such as video games or television. While these pastimes may

---

[52] Blasingame, G. (2001). Developmentally disabled sexual offender rehavilitative treatment program manual and form. *Wood 'N' Barnes Publishing*.

serve to distract you from your urges, you can only move beyond those urges by actively cultivating a sense of purpose and accomplishment. There are three categories in particular that you should focus on—and generally in this order.

Physical fitness. Idle hands and minds invite temptations, so exercise is an important resource in your metaphorical toolbox; not only does it serve as a great outlet for excess energy, but when done right exercise will also improve your health, mood, and self-confidence. We are more vulnerable to relapse when feeling bad, and regular exercise has been shown to be just as effective as antidepressants in treating clinical depression,[53] perhaps in part because aerobic conditioning increases the number of D_2 dopamine receptors in the brain.[54] Exercise outside whenever possible. Sunlight has been shown to benefit health and mood as well,[55] so you might as well combine the two. Select exercises that you enjoy (or can come to enjoy) and that you can see being a long-term part of your life. If you are new to physical fitness, experiment. Ask friends for help or sign up for classes. Some find that meditation in conjunction with yoga, which strives to discipline both the body and the mind, helps them to achieve the self-awareness and self-control that is so valuable to this journey.

As important to physical and mental fitness as exercise is the fuel we put inside of our bodies. Improper foods can deplete our energy levels, harm our health, and lower our mood. Healthful foods can fill us with energy and motivation. In an era of thousands of competing opinions it can be difficult to know what food is healthy, so do your own research. In general, avoid heavily processed foods in favor of whole foods close to how they appear in nature—fruits, vegetables, whole grains, nuts, and seeds.

Passions and purpose. PMO tends to nudge aside more healthy hobbies to make room for itself, so now that you are recovering you may discover more free time. Since sitting alone in your room wondering what to do invites temptation, it is time to rediscover and

[53] Blumenthal, J., Babyak, M., Moore K., et al. (1999). Effects of exercise training on older patients with major depression. *Arch Intern Med*, 159(19), 2349-2356.

[54] MacRae, P., Spirduso, W., Cartee, G., Farrar, R., Wilcox, R. (1987, August 18). Endurance training effects on striatal D2 dopamine receptor binding and striatal dopamine metabolite levels. *National Center for Biotechnology Information*. Web.

[55] Edwards, L., & Torcellini, P. (2002, July). A literature review of the effects of natural light on building occupants. Web.

reignite your passions. Passions are those activities and pursuits that fascinate and challenge you. Passions are what can fill your hours and leave you with a sense of pride rather than a sense of emptiness. Passions are what you talk to people about at dinner parties. Re-watching old episodes of *M.A.S.H.* or going for your highest kill streak on *Call of Duty* are not passions. Music, juggling, spelunking, coaching football, classic blender restoration—these are passions. Find yours and pursue them, but also recognize that they are side dishes. Passions are yummy and can make an underwhelming entree more palatable, but to find true satisfaction we need purpose.

Whether you are a 20-something man-child living with his parents or a middle-aged middle-manager questioning the 30 years he dedicated to his corporate masters, almost every man can benefit from being more in touch with his personal mission, especially if he has no idea what that mission is. Do not gloss over this step, as this is the step most likely to help you succeed in this journey and in your life. If you already know what your purpose is (i.e. start a business, pursue art, save the whales, save the whaling industry) then there is no better time than now to throw yourself into that pursuit. You have all that free time since you quit PMO—use it wisely. The more you accomplish with this time, the stronger you will feel and the farther away you will be from relapsing and returning to your old life.

If you do not know what you want out of this life, you must figure it out. No one can do this for you. The best piece of counsel I can give is as cliché as it is true: follow your heart. Family, society, and friends have all conditioned you to remain on the path carved out by their expectations. This is usually the "safe" path (though in truth it is anything but). Your parents want you to get a degree and secure a place on the corporate ladder—and be sure it provides dental. Society wants you to accrue volunteer hours and internships to pad your resumé and impress your betters. Your friends want you to toe the line so that they are not forced to reconsider their own lives. But none of them is in a position to know what is right for you.

The truth is that your head probably does not know what is right for you, either, which is why you must listen to your body—your heart. When confronted with a life-altering choice, close your eyes and visualize each option one at a time. Imagine the years ahead of you and how they may play out given each path. As you visualize, remain aware of how your body reacts. Do you feel signs of resistance, such as scrunching shoulders, a frown, or a wrinkling brow? Or do you feel a smile and easy breathing? The body can let the mind know what the heart wants—if you pay attention. The precise physical signs vary from individual to individual, but the principle applies to everyone. You can feel the right choice.

If you have no options to consider or all of them are shoulder-scrunchers, then you really must just start living. Experiment. Try new things. Make new friends. Read prolifically. Use the Internet to research something other than your favorite porn stars. Simply put, live as much as possible until you encounter that which feels right, and then heed that feeling.

If you need more guidance, there is an exercise you may find helpful, but like everything else in this book you have to commit to it to reap the reward. Write, "What is the purpose of my life?" Write your answer. When finished, write another answer, something completely different or a revision of what you wrote before. Repeat. Continue repeating until you write the answer that makes you cry. This answer expresses your true purpose as you feel it now.

Social skills. It is time to break out of your cocoon, little butterfly. Once you have improved your self-assurance by taking charge of your body and your life, it is time to share the new you with the world. Whatever your previous level of social acumen, undertaking this journey will likely increase both your ability and your motivation to enjoy time with others. As the weeks go by without artificial fulfillment of sexual and emotional needs, many previous introverts or reluctant extroverts find themselves powerfully motivated to become more social creatures. Now that you are filling your time with healthy and heartfelt pursuits, you will have plenty to talk about. And now that you are free of shame and comfortable sharing your story with others, you will become fearless and commanding in conversation. Enjoy it.

However, whether your goal is to meet new romantic partners or friends, know that you can only foster deep connections with others if you are willing to expose your vulnerabilities. The more people you allow to accept you for who you are, the less shame will hold you down and the stronger you will be at pursuing your new life. Perhaps your opening line should not be, "I'm addicted to tranny porn", but if porn use and recovery is an important part of your life at the moment, then you should share it at some point.

11. Rewire. In the reboot you allow your body to clear the neurophysiologic slate of porn's presence. Now you need to fill that slate up with what you really want to enjoy. For most men this is natural, loving sex with their chosen partners, free from worry about sexual dysfunction or emotional disconnect due to porn-induced desensitization. For this to happen, you must "rewire" with a partner. Have fun. Explore your partner. Talk openly about your feelings concerning sex. Take it slowly if you feel the need. A big part of rewiring is simply being close with your partner, cuddling, kissing, and associating warm, sexual feelings with his or her presence. Over time you will condition your sexual response system to react to genuine rather than artificial stimuli, and real sex should only continue to get easier and better for you.

Knowing when to start having sex again is difficult, and each man must experiment and find the timetable that works best for him. You can skip the reboot entirely, in fact. Just stop using PMO and/or MO, continue to have sex, and see what happens. If you suffer from sexual dysfunction or believe that you are not enjoying sex as much as you should, however, then you may need a deliberate period of rest in order to re-sensitize your sexual response system. Know that continuing to have sex and reach orgasm soon after quitting PMO may slow this healing process considerably. Additionally, if you are accustomed to frequent sexual release, then this period of complete abstinence will show you that you can live without indulging lust.

Depending on the depth and consistency of your PMO abuse, you may need a longer or shorter reboot before you feel ready to rewire. Older men especially find that they need less reboot time in order to return to the sexual pathways they wired in their youth—approximately one or two months. Younger men who grew up on porn or who started using PMO before having real sex may need much longer. Many encounter success with 90 days, but you may need half of a year or more—or less. I recommend a minimum of 30 days without sexual release for all men on this journey. If you suffer from PIED and want to see a specific physical sign of recovery before trying to have sex, wait until you get strong erections just from passionate kissing.

If you already have a romantic partner, then the rewire becomes much easier. As I recommended in "share", you should keep your partner completely updated on your journey. The only way that he or she can fully help you is if you are open about the intimacies of your struggle. Make sure to stress that rewiring is a process, that whatever problems you are trying to heal will still take time to completely surpass but that you are committed to attaining a healthier, more enjoyable love life no matter how long it takes. What you want to accomplish with this conversation is to limit expectations; if you do not, then expectations may end up limiting you. This is especially true for men with PIED. Since PIED feeds performance anxiety and vice versa, you may still have trouble getting and maintaining an erection after a reboot simply because you are anxious about the results, wondering what will happen and checking your erection rather than enjoying the moment and focusing on exploring your partner. Instead, do not worry about your erection or reaching orgasm. Know that it will happen eventually and that there is no need to rush it. Just have fun.

If you have DE or desensitization or your libido is greatly decreased over the days following orgasm, then you should not use your hands to "finish yourself off" during sex. Often recovering sufferers of PIDE can get close to orgasm during sex but need to manually stimulate themselves in order to go over the edge. In this case, you are not truly ready for orgasm. If you cannot reach climax solely with the touch of a partner, then do not climax. This may take some willpower in the moment, but it will cue your body that sensitivity needs to increase in order to orgasm. If you cheat yourself by using your own hand, then you send the "good enough" signal to stop re-sensitizing and adapting to another's touch.

Additionally, some men find that frequent orgasm with a partner (especially during the first few months of their recovery) drains them of focus, energy, and libido—or it intensifies cravings for PMO in what is called the "chaser effect". These men may benefit from using *coitus reservatus* or "karezza", which simply refers to sex without orgasm and often results in slower, longer, more affectionate, less frantic lovemaking, with the man remaining at a sustainable level of pleasure (not repeatedly approaching and retreating from orgasm).

12. You may have noticed that the most important step has so far been left out of this list, but that is because each item above embodies it. The twelfth step is to **commit** to your new life. With the completion of each step, you are **committing** further and further to this journey. This commitment will shape your new reality. Several weeks or months from now, each day free from PMO and more engaged with real opportunities will feel natural to you, and you will wonder how you ever could have been the person you were just a short time ago. You will realize that a porn-free life is not something dreadful that you must nonetheless embrace for your sexual health; it is in fact a wonderful, awesome prospect that excites you more with each passing day.

Understand that this commitment must exist at a deeper level than you are used to. You have probably "committed" to endeavors in the past that you failed, but those were not true commitments. Those were goals, and goals can be missed. So do not think of this journey as a goal. To help illustrate this concept, imagine cutting off your own hand with a hatchet. The thought of doing this repels you because it would cause you regret and pain and would inflict lasting damage upon your lifestyle. Do you have to fight urges to cut off your hand? No! The possibility might come into your mind once in a while because humans are zany creatures who have weird thoughts, but you do not have to struggle with this decision because it is *not really a decision*. Cutting off your own hand exists outside the realm of possibility for you, so it is not worth more than a passing thought. The same must be true of PMO. You do not set a goal to avoid cutting off your hand for 90 days; it is simply a fact of your underlying reality.

This is an extreme comparison, yes, but if you need this guide then PMO use also causes you regret and pain and inflicts lasting damage upon your lifestyle, so there is no reason that it should be a possibility for you. I hope that the thought of battling urges to cut off your hand made you chuckle, because it is funny. Adopt the same sense of humor about PMO. Once you master this level of commitment, you should not have to battle urges to use. You battle opponents you respect; opponents have a chance of winning. PMO has no chance, so you laugh it off.

This list is designed to give you the best possible opportunity to heal yourself. That said, this is not a homework assignment. This is your life. Only you are in charge of your journey. There is no one right way to do this, and there are men who have successfully healed themselves without completing one or more of these steps—only you can decide what is right for you. Each addict is addicted to a varying degree, and some will be able to free themselves more easily and casually than others. Before you decide against completing any of these steps, however, ask yourself whether your decision to skip it is determined by fear: fear of commitment, shame, embarrassment, change, etc. If the answer is yes, then you are allowing fear to dictate your life. You have to decide if you can accept that.

13. Relapse: the sometimes-necessary 13th step. It is said that we learn more from our failures than from our successes, and that is how you should choose to look at relapse if it happens. Some amount of relapsing usually occurs while quitting PMO, but it is possible to turn such a stumble into a leap forward. A relapse despite your best efforts can teach you many things: how strong your addiction is, what your triggers are, how your mind rationalizes PMO use, how you react emotionally to a relapse, etc.

The first step in dealing with a relapse is to forgive yourself. Regret the mistake, but do not regret who you are, for it is human to make mistakes. If instead you tell yourself that you are weak and a failure, then you are much more likely to use again in order to dull the pain of self-loathing. Second, analyze critically how it happened, why it happened, and how you feel about it. Was it satisfying to you? Was it as good as you hoped it would be? Do you want to continue doing it? Then plan for the future, deciding how you will better avoid triggers and deal with urges. Again, do not dwell on failure; this increases the urge to make yourself feel better by giving in again ("I've already failed so what the hell, I may as well enjoy it"). Instead, be content with the new knowledge you have acquired and get excited about how it will help you to accomplish your goals.

If you continuously relapse, however, then you must consider the possibility that you are not ready to live without PMO. If so, stop trying to quit for awhile. Enjoy your PMO sessions and then move on, as berating yourself afterward only brings more negative energy into your life. Instead, just channel your focus into something productive that you are passionate about. Reread the "fill the void" section of this guide. After enough time enhancing the positive aspects of your life, you may find yourself strong and confident enough to move on from PMO.

If the proposition of delaying your new, PMO-free life even for that long disgusts you, however, then I have some more tactics for you. Each tactic is a tool in your willpower toolbox that, if used properly, can help you become the person you want to be. Instead of trying to employ all of them at once, focus and commit to one or two at a time in order to fairly evaluate its value in your own journey.

Free yourself of shame. If you need this section then I must repeat myself. Research professor Brené Brown spent six years studying shame and how it plays into our choices, our relationships, and our happiness. According to Brown, "Guilt: 'Sorry, I made a mistake.' Shame: 'Sorry, I *am* a mistake.' [...] Shame is highly, highly correlated with addiction, depression, violence, aggression, bullying, suicide, eating disorders. And here's what you even need to know more: guilt—

inversely correlated with those things."[56] Guilt is what we feel after making a choice that goes against our ideals. Shame is what we feel when we believe that we are fundamentally bad, unsalvageable. Guilt is a powerful tool that drives us toward being the person we want to be. Shame is an anchor. You can and should let go of that anchor. You are not your choices nor your mistakes, so do not despise yourself for your mistakes—despise your mistakes for yourself.

Reframe your reality. We humans tend to want to hold onto what we have. Losing what we already see as ours hurts more than receiving something new helps, even if there is a rational net gain. So visualize yourself months from now and free of addiction, enjoying the benefits of recovery and the resolution of whatever problems brought you to this guide. You are happier, healthier, and more productive than ever before. Now accept that this future is what will happen—it is yours to lose. No one can take it from you but yourself. "I have to give up PMO in order to have a brighter future" becomes "I would have to give up my bright future in order to PMO." Sound like a worthy trade?

Cultivate mindfulness. There are two main parts of our brains that we are interested in for the purposes of examining willpower. We have the limbic system, which you should already know plenty about. It is the older and baser system for regulating desire and motivation. This is where our urges and cravings come from. Then we have the prefrontal cortex, which is where our restraint, goal setting, and long-term decision making come into play. If not for this part of our brains, we would act on all of our baser, momentary inclinations and have no grasp on the grander direction we would like our lives to take. When you hold yourself back from eating the last three slices of cake, that is your prefrontal cortex at work.

Thanks to the gift of neuroplasticity, just as you can strengthen and grow the parts of your brain that control motor and visual functions by juggling, so too can you strengthen the parts of your brain that govern willpower and high-level decision making. This can be especially important since addiction tends to weaken and atrophy those brain regions ("hypofrontality"). Instead of juggling, though, you must practice mindfulness.

We make the majority of our decisions on autopilot; our conscious minds do not even recognize that there is a decision to be made. When

---

[56] Brown, B. (2012, March). Listening to shame. *TED.* Web.

most people check Facebook, take a second helping of gravy, or press the snooze button, they are not consciously deciding to do so—they just follow an urge. Our limbic systems want social acceptance, fatty foods, and sleep, and this is good because all of them are beneficial in the right amounts. But because we live in a modern environment where overindulgence is a constant danger, we have to train our conscious minds to monitor those urges and make the final call about whether we truly want these things right now or if they are getting in the way of our grander commitments (being less distracted at work, losing weight, developing a morning routine, etc.). The way we train this skill is by consistently reminding ourselves to be conscious of our thoughts and actions.

Carry a piece of paper and pen with you. Whenever it comes time to make a willpower decision concerning your addiction (or anything else you would like to be more mindful of), write down your choices. This will likely have something to do with your triggers, such as "Watch video of Miami Dolphins cheerleaders covering 'Call Me Maybe' vs. go for a run." Circle the choice that you make, then do it. This simple practice activates your conscious decision-making ability, which—once activated—can easily override your unwanted urges. Just seeing those two choices opposed in writing will, more often than not, allow you to make the right choice for your long-term aspirations.

Once you practice this technique enough, you can just verbalize the choices to yourself rather than bothering with writing them down, but starting with pen and paper will give you a product at the end of the day that you can look back to proudly or as a learning experience.

If you do circle the choice that aligns with your unwanted temptation, then narrate your thought process out loud as you follow through with that decision. This will keep the prefrontal cortex activated and give you as many opportunities as possible to intervene and set yourself back on the right track. For example, as I am clicking on the video I might say, "I am fully aware that the Miami Dolphins cheerleaders are one sexy group of women and that I am clicking on this link just because of my sexual desire to see them. Watching this video goes against my commitment not to get turned on by pixels and will probably lead to me masturbating furiously to bukkake porn. I have been experiencing some really good progress lately, and this choice jeopardizes those gains. I should at least take a few minutes outside to breathe deeply and think about this some more." You get the idea. If you use this technique to maintain mindfulness, your chances are greatly increased of making the decision that is right for your long-term hopes and commitments.

Accept your thoughts, control your actions. Part of cultivating mindfulness is learning to watch our own thoughts without trying to control or banish them. If I tell you that you absolutely cannot think about elephants for the next five minutes, you will be thinking about elephants constantly; banishing thoughts with brute force like this not only does not work but produces the opposite effect. Similarly, if I tell you that it is of vital importance that you not look at porn for the next month, you will constantly be thinking about porn. And the more you tell yourself not to think about it, the more it will pop into your mind. Your fear of cravings gives those cravings power over you.

Instead, when a craving or thought about using rises, just breathe and observe your own mind and body. The monster under the bed only has power when the lights are off, so turn on the floodlights, flip the bed over, and look the monster in the eye. Accept that you are having these thoughts and feelings, examine them like a scientist studying wildlife. Watch as the craving gets stronger, and keep watching as it gets weaker and flickers out. The monster *will* look away first. This process will teach you that your cravings do not control you. You do not even need to fight urges; just watch them until they subside, realizing that your cravings do not control your actions: *you do.*

This technique takes a few tries to get good at, so practice and perfect it on less consequential cravings such as scratching an itch on your nose or eating the last slice of pizza.

Meditate. A proven way to strengthen your mindfulness muscles is through breath meditation.[57] For as little as five minutes each day, sit in a comfortable position, close your eyes, and focus on the sensation of your breath. Do not try to control it. Just observe and feel the inhalations and exhalations. If you notice other thoughts popping into your head or your attention wandering, simply take note of it and shift your focus back to the breath. Do not get angry at yourself for slipping or try to push these thoughts away. The goal of this practice is not to maintain a blissfully clear mind, but to notice when your thoughts wander and to nudge your focus back into line. Each time this happens is a victory that activates and exercises the prefrontal cortex, preparing it to notice and interrupt cravings that you would prefer not to satisfy.

---

[57] Cromie, W. (2006, February 2). Meditation found to increase brain size. *Harvard Gazette*. Web.

Take 10 minutes. Sometimes the prospect of abstaining from PMO for life, for 90 days, or even for a day can seem overwhelming. So when you feel like you absolutely have to look at porn or masturbate, just abstain for 10 minutes. Take 10 minutes, then allow yourself the choice again. Ideally, you should use those 10 minutes to move yourself to a different environment, breathe, reactivate your mindfulness, remind yourself of your goals, and then start another activity.

When the 10 minutes is up, you may find that the craving has dissipated and you do not need to relapse anymore. Or you may still want to relapse but can give it another 10 minutes, and then maybe another 10 after that, and then it is time for dinner and you forget all about it. Or maybe you do give in after the 10 minutes, but at least you gave it 10 minutes, and that is a lot better than what you used to do. If you cannot last through the first 10 minutes, then that should raise a red flag for you: your addiction is so strong that you could not control it for even a few moments.

The 10 minutes tactic can also help you to engage in positive activities (it has been vital in helping me to overcome procrastination). If there is something you should be doing but you are tempted to procrastinate, just work on what needs to be done for 10 minutes before allowing yourself the option to slack off. By the end of 10 minutes, you may be on a roll and not want to stop—or at least be willing to give it another 10 minutes.

Extinguish triggers. If you find that the triggers you cannot avoid are overpowering you, you can take away their power by repeatedly confronting them in a controlled manner. If you are triggered by the address bar in a web browser, for example, type in the address of a favorite porn site. Stay in the moment and be mindful of how this makes you feel, then delete the address. Do this many times over many days and your brain will adapt to dismiss the former trigger instead of expecting PMO to follow. If you are afraid that you will just give in to the urge rather than breaking the cycle, first try this in a safe environment such as in public or with a friend present.

Raise the stakes. In the heat of the moment, it can be all too easy to forget why it is important not to just give in, so make it important enough that you cannot forget. For example, identify a charity, cause, or political party that goes against everything you believe in. Donate $100 to it every time you relapse, no exceptions. Soon you will be laughing off your cravings like a boss. Or you will be explaining to your friends why you have donated thousands to the American Nazi Party.

Change your environment. More than we like to admit, we are products of our environment, heavily influenced by our friends, popular media, and old habits. And an environment has inertia. Like the human brain, the little world each of us lives in settles into a certain way of doing things, and to resist this momentum is like swimming upstream: usually doable but very difficult. If you need to transform your life, sometimes it is easier just to get out of the stream and walk somewhere else.

You can change your environment in small ways, such as moving your computer to a more public location or placing cues for positive activities around your home. But you can also change your environment in drastic ways. It might not be so hard to resist PMO when you are backpacking across Iceland with no electronic devices but a GPS, volunteering for the Peace Corps in South America, or going through boot camp for the armed services. Thrust yourself into a drastically unfamiliar situation and you will be far too busy surviving to obsess over your no-PMO streak. Before you know it you will have moved on with your life. Just be wary to not return to bad old habits when you return to an old environment.

Lighten up. It is easy to become exhausted if you feel as though you constantly have to resist urges, but the beautiful and horrible truth about our own unwanted cravings is that they only have as much power as we give them. If you fear relapse then you allow for the possibility of relapse. If you fight urges as though they are opponents, then you give them a chance at victory. Instead, trust yourself. Decide to change and know with that it will happen. You have complete control over this change, so there is no reason to doubt its certainty—it is not as if someone will force you to relapse. Once you trust yourself, urges are more like crickets chirping at your feet than formidable opponents. They are noticeable, but all they can make you do is smile in amusement as you move on with your life. When you wake up in the morning and the thought of relapse crosses your mind, laugh, shake your head at the funny joke, and go make yourself some oatmeal.

Read *The Willpower Instinct* by Kelly McGonagall. It is the most helpful text on willpower that I have found, and several of these tactics are inspired by McGonagall's research. I do not receive any advertising kickbacks from recommending it (but if you would like to start, Kelly, give me a call).

My Story

You know how I began this journey. Here I include a selection of my online journal entries over the next several months in order to provide an in-depth example of one man's recovery: my own.

Day 1 — Mood: 6/10 — Libido: 0/10

After researching my problems further and discovering that they were caused by porn addiction, felt zero sexual urge of any kind. Very introspective. Started writing my story, didn't stop till exhausted. I don't see myself having any urges in the future to watch porn after what I've realized it's done to me, but neither will I get complacent.

Day 2 — Mood: 6/10 — Libido: 2/10

Woke up from a nap twice to notice that I was erect. Squeezed my Kegels a few times and felt good, but otherwise ignored it. Wrote for most of the rest of the day and into the night. I need to get this all down. Maybe it can help others but at the very least it will help me purge and understand myself.

Day 3 — Mood: 5/10 — Libido: 3/10

For awhile in the morning I found it difficult to keep recent romantic memories out of my head, and I definitely felt some stirring, but I didn't indulge, and at least I was remembering real experiences with a real woman rather than pornography. Finished writing my sexual story up till now. Will post it tonight. I feel a bit let down, but I think that's natural after finishing with something that has so thoroughly swept me away.

There is a woman I recently met whom I've been on two dates with. We are very compatible and I like her a lot. The timing of us meeting is strange, though, as you all can tell from my story. What I need most right now is to heal myself of my addiction and be honest with people, so I'm going to tell her the basics of this tomorrow. If that doesn't scare her off, I'll direct her here to read my entire story. Woman I've Been On Two Dates With, I totally understand if all this freaks you out and you want no part of my burdens, but I really, really don't want another relationship with a woman in which I am silent and keeping secrets, so I'm sharing this with you. At the least I hope you've learned a lot about the modern technology-age man (unfortunately it's all scary and ****ed up). If you're not scared away, I do like you and would like to continue getting to know you better, but you should know that I won't be ready to be a fully functional male companion for any woman for at least a couple of months (a guess according to my reading of other men's accounts).

Day 4 — Mood: 9/10 — Libido: 5/10

Woman I've Been On Two Dates With is now Woman I've Been On Three Dates With, but that name seems a little long. Let's call her Erika. We went on a long run today, and I told her about the basics of my porn addiction, sexual difficulties, and commitment to a period of complete abstinence in order to do something about it. It was so easy. I truly do feel like a different person than I was a couple of months ago.

She was not scared away, and I told her that I had spent the last 3 days writing the whole story and had posted it to this forum. I said that she could read it if she wanted but it contained my entire sexual history and maybe she didn't want to know me quite this well yet. She agreed. She seemed very pleased that I had told her everything, though, and she said it was partly a relief because she is a virgin (which I knew) and feared that I was just interested in her for sex. Maybe we met at just the right time.

We spent about 5 hours together, some of it on the couch exploring each other a bit while fully clothed. I had a partial-to-full erection for some of this time, and after she left the blue balls set in. Oh well :)

Soon after she left, she texted me saying that she had been thinking about it and was very curious to read my story, so I sent it to her. I was 100% sure that being open about everything was the right thing to do, and I was well prepared for her to not want to see me again after reading the details. Nevertheless I can admit that I was still a little worried. A few hours later, I found a very sweet message from her on Facebook. She says that she is grateful for my trust in sharing this with her and would also very much like to get to know me better. She tells me to take all the time I need to heal, and that she would like to develop a trusting and committed relationship before having sex for the first time anyway.

I am very happy with my new honest self and honest relationship :) If anyone out there is keeping secrets like this that he would like to share with the people in his life, I recommend it. A life lived honestly and openly is so much more fulfilling. Mood: 9/10

Day 5 — Mood: 8/10 — Libido: 3/10

After work, told my best friend all about this. Easy. He was especially interested because he thinks that porn addiction may have had negative effects on his life as well, though he has had fulfilling sexual relationships. We went to this Lebanese restaurant where there was a pretty server he wanted to see more of, and I encouraged him to get her number. He was a bit nervous about it, but things like this seem like no big deal to me anymore. There was another pretty server there, and I thought it would be easy to get her contact and connect later, but I'd like to see where things are going with Erika right now.

Day 8 — Mood: 6/10 — Libido: 4/10

Since I have given up P and most movies and TV, I have been accomplishing quite a bit more. I am strongly considering writing a book about high-speed Internet porn addiction that will include my (hopefully) successful story and some of the stories of people in this community who would like to share with a greater audience.

Best friend decided to give up porn indefinitely and abstain from M for at least awhile. He says that he feels 5x more productive since abstaining (he's usually a daily Mer). Two other friends have also committed to giving up P since I've shared this info with them.

I am very curious to experience my changing physical and emotional states as I go through this process over the next year. So far this hasn't been difficult, but I know from many men's accounts that flatline and depression often occur after the initial short-term euphoria of commitment.

Days 9, 10 — Mood: 8/10 — Libido: 2/10

Wow, this is an amazing experience. I almost cannot believe the positive changes that have occurred in my life over the last weeks. If you read my first post, you know that these changes began before learning about arousal addiction, so I can't give all the credit to stopping PMO, but it is certainly a big part of it.

During my waking hours, I've seldom been more focused, creative, and excited to work. Ideas for projects to work on and plans for my future are just easily flowing into me, and I'm having very little of my old troubles with laziness and procrastination. Social anxiety is almost totally gone, which is especially noticeable on the phone. I used to dread phone calls because I wasn't sure I could fill the silence and it would become awkward, but now they're fun, and I'm excited to connect with people. Again, I can't give complete credit to no PMO for this change, but it's certainly contributing. And before anyone smacks down my good vibe, I know that I am likely to experience depression and bad times once this initial euphoria is over, but I do think that this is part of a lasting upswing.

Of course, not everything is great. I should note that my "libido" rating each day refers to my physical libido—how my penis feels about women and sex. Unless I'm going through some serious emotional turmoil, my mind is pretty much always very interested. This is especially true right now, but I can definitely tell that my body is not ready yet. I have read that it often takes 90 days of a complete-abstinence reboot to heal enough for an effective rewire with a woman. Though after 90 days I may masturbate once to sensation (no fantasy) to test myself, really I have very little desire to masturbate again. Like, ever. We'll see how my feelings about that evolve. Erika and I are still seeing each other, by the way. The other day she commented that she feels we've known each other a lot longer than two weeks, and I agreed. When you're really open and honest with someone, it's amazing how close you can become in a short time. Anyway, it's going to be tough to be patient over the next few months, but I suppose I have plenty of other things to do in the meantime.

I am doing one thing right that I think is really important. Anytime I see something on a screen that arouses me at all, I close it or walk away. This includes FB pics, hot dancers in music videos, etc. Obviously I haven't been watching much, but I think this is important. Allowing myself any leeway could easily lead too far (oh I'll just look up some pics of that actress...). Also, my laptop does not ever go into my room anymore, as there is no need to tempt myself by having it next to my bed as usual.

Days 11, 12 — Mood: 5/10 — Libido: 3/10

I've had a few more intense cravings for particularly memorable porn scenes or porn stars. They are still nowhere near as powerful as my reasons for quitting, but they can be surprisingly strong.

My dreams are definitely more intense than they used to be. Every other night or so there is one about porn, but mostly they are just more involved and memorable than they have been for quite awhile. I may start keeping a dream journal again.

Day 20 — Mood: 6/10 — Libido: 5/10

Life is busy. This is good. Pornography rarely comes to mind anymore, and though fantasies still come into my head, they are first-person fantasies about real women in my life—not porn re-creations. I am having more dreams about sex, though no wet dreams so far (I've never had one).

Day 22 — Mood: 8/10 — Libido: 8/10

Spent some more time in bed today with Erika, and ended up dry humping fully hard with her for about ten minutes. It felt good. It felt like having sex would be the most natural thing in the world. I felt ready. I used to dread sex I knew it probably wouldn't go well, but now I'm looking forward to it. I don't know how far along the healing process I am or how these feelings will change from here, but I know I'm in a better place than I've been in a long time.

My friend had sex for the first time since no PMO, and he says he was much more passionate than usual, and it was much more enjoyable.

Day 25 — Mood: 8/10 — Libido: 6/10

In the evening, I hopped on my motorcycle and rode the 25 miles to Erika's house for the first time. I met her family (who left soon after for a party) and we spent the evening making dinner, relaxing in her sauna, and playing around. I was hard several times, but the feeling wasn't quite as strong as a few days ago, which made me question if I am ready for sex. I know that most men like me aren't feeling the full effects of the healing process until 90 days in, and I am only on day 25. I won't be embarrassed in front of Erika if we try and I am not ready, but I just don't want to experience that again. What do you guys think?

I left just after 11 and cruised down pitch-black country highways at 70 mph in near-freezing temperatures. There's no feeling like it. I realize that I am happy. This month has had plenty of ups and downs, but I know I'm heading in the right direction, and life is just so much fun. I'm never going back.

Day 28 — Mood: 5/10 — Libido: 7/10

Despite waking up with wood every day, I've started to feel like my libido is going down because sexual thoughts are coming into my mind less and less. But then today while out in town I no more than walked past an attractive woman and all of that energy that I thought was missing was suddenly very present. I was half hard very quickly and felt a pressing need for her. This must mean that my libido is transferring away from fantasy and back toward real, present women, and the feeling was good.

Day 30 — Mood: 6/10 — Libido: 6/10

This is it, boys, 30 days in! I can safely say that this is the longest I have gone without masturbation and orgasm in my entire life, probably since about age 2-3. I'm in truly uncharted territory now, and there's no turning back.

Day 35 — Mood: 7/10 — Libido: 7/10

Erika ended up in my bed again today. I've never experienced such a slow, passionate sexual progression before—not even with Amy, my first serious girlfriend. Each time we go a little further, discovering a little bit more of each other, and we appreciate every moment in its every sensual detail.

Today we were dry humping in various positions in our underwear for at least a half hour, and I was fully hard for most of the time. Later, I guided her hand down and she started to massage my penis. I've never been able to get much pleasure from a handjob—I much prefer oral—but this felt better than I remembered. I still lost my erection a bit though, partly because I think I'm still regaining sensitivity and partly because the head of my dick hurt from grinding against the inside of my underwear for a half hour. A little while later she asked if I had a condom. I did. I asked if she wanted to have sex. She said yes.

I thought for a moment, then told her, "Not yet." It didn't feel like the right time. Aside from already having friction burns on my penis and blue balls due to over an hour of teasing, I want to explore manual and oral sex more first. I want to experience those sensations with a lasting erection and perhaps reach O with a partner at least once before we try having sex. I feel like that will go a long way toward ridding me of any lingering anxiety caused by PIED. Plus, I'm only 35 days in. I've made leagues of progress from where I was, but I feel like there are still many leagues ahead before I'm at full sexual function. I'm really enjoying this slow build of our sexual relationship and don't feel like it's time for the climax yet (figuratively or literally). It's strange, but I don't feel compelled to rush this. Though going as slow as we are is equal parts torturous and intoxicating, it feels right for now.

Erika told me to take as long as I need, and she meant it. I'm happy she's with me. Though I can tell that she's definitely feeling the torturous part. She told me that she's woken up wet every morning this week and masturbated thinking about me. No one has ever said *that* to me before. ****ing hot.

Day 36 — Mood: 6/10 — Libido: N/A

I've realized that my libido measure isn't very productive. You'd think that a higher number is better, right? But this journey has taught me that I shouldn't have and don't want a noticeably high libido every day. I think that a natural sex drive is a subtle undercurrent of energy most of the time. It infuses me with motivation and focus, and it lets me direct that energy how I so choose. Only when I encounter a real, attractive woman should it come into its own and manifest in a sexual lust. My life determines my libido; my libido does not determine my life. At least that's how I feel I'm becoming. So the libidometer is changing. On days like today it will read "N/A" (not applicable). I didn't feel much lust or strong urges for sex, but does that mean I had a low libido? No. It was there, waiting. On days when it should express itself, I'll still rate from 1-10 on how strongly it manifests and how well I am able to use it.

Day 45 — Mood: 7/10 — Libido: 8/10

Valentine's Day. I usually only write about Erika in relation to my sexual progress. I do this because this is a journal about sex, but I'd like to say that I care for her and I'm very glad that she's in my life not just because she's helping me rewire.

I have made so much progress with my PIED. Today as Erika and I were cutting fruit, we held hands for a moment, and just the feel of our hands together slippery with fruit juice caused me to get fully hard—I got a full erection from holding hands. Words cannot express how glad I am that I decided to undertake this journey, for this reason and many others. Stay strong, brothers.

Day 58 — Mood: 5/10 — Libido: N/A

It's been a couple of weeks since I've journalled, and that's because there hasn't been much to write about in this aspect of my life. I feel like my libido has taken a downswing. For awhile I had this barely dormant sexual energy and would get erect from a memory or a slight real-life stimulus, but that's receded. Sometimes I felt this buildup inside of me and feel like I was about to orgasm while limp and doing nothing, but that's gone too. I can't really call this a flatline because I get morning wood every day and get hard with Erika, but it doesn't last as long as a few weeks ago, and if I'm not with her I don't feel any sexual urges. Maybe this is my flatline. I really have no idea what comes next. There is that question in my mind: "Is this it?" Intellectually I know (and hope) that the answer is "no". I know that many men have taken much longer than 60 days to feel recovered, and I know that recovery is not linear, but it's disheartening nonetheless. All I really know is that it's been two months since P, M, or O for me. And in regards to M and O, that's one month longer than any other time in my life since before I can remember (2-3 years old). It's like walking down a path blindfolded, but I'll keep putting one foot in front of the other and have faith in a better tomorrow. Crossing my fingers.

Other parts of my life are going well. Erika and I are "Facebook official" now, and I really enjoy being with her. We've been doing a lot of acroyoga, in which I basically lift her into the air in various ways, lol. It's really fun, and I recommend it for anybody with a SO on here. I've started a new weightlifting cycle with a friend, and I'm expecting big gains. I'm volunteering with an organization that I really believe in, and I think I can do some good. I've been a vegan for over four years, and I've begun transitioning to a raw food lifestyle, which is something I've wanted to do for awhile. Professionally, I'm basically investing all of my time into an entrepreneurial project, hoping that I don't run out of money before I get it off the ground and the season for my summer job starts.

Hope I have more to journal about soon—

Days 65-69 — Mood: ranging from 3-9/10 — Libido: ranging from 1-9/10

Whew, what a weekend. As you can see, it went from quite bad to very good and everywhere in between. Libido felt like it was back on an upswing at the beginning of the week; my penis stopped feeling like it was trying to hide from something and regained its (flaccid) fullness. On Thursday, Erika tried giving head for the first time. She's a quick learner, and it felt great, but I wasn't fully hard for a lot of it. After taking a break so I could play with her for awhile, I was down and not coming back up. I realized later that this was because I was in the beginning stages of what would soon become a 103 degree fever, during which I had absolutely zero sex urge. I was planning on spending the weekend with my parents anyway, so I went there to rest up. Erika came by a lot to bring me food and take care of me—she's awesome.

My mom also took care of me. She's great at that. I still haven't told my parents about all this, though I plan to. I know they're wondering what all is going on in my life right now since I am spending a lot of time writing a book about this, and I would like to tell them, but something is impelling me to wait. I think it's pride. I'll tell any curious stranger off the street all about the whole journey, porn addiction, etc. because the opinions of strangers mean nothing to me, but I hate having to disappoint and upset my parents, because I love them. I know that hearing I've been a porn addict since 9 years old won't be easy for my mom especially, and I'd like to tell them after I've succeeded in the journey and am close to finishing the book, so that at least I can show them that I've transformed something dark into something positive that could help others. Maybe that's wrong and I should tell them now, but...I don't want to. Not yet.

On Sunday night, I was with Erika in my room at my parents' house. I looked into her eyes and I just felt this really strong need to tell her that I love her.

I've only said that to one other woman, and I didn't really mean it then. I was in high school, I was numbed from PMO, I didn't know what love really felt like, and I said it because she said it to me. I ended up breaking her heart, and I promised that I wouldn't say it again unless I really felt it.

But I felt it on Sunday, so I told Erika that I love her. Wow. I wasn't sure that I would ever feel that! Did I not feel it for such a long time in my life because I was numbed by PMO, or because I hadn't met the right woman, or because I wasn't in an honest relationship? All three, I think.

And if you're wondering, yes, she said it back...but I've known for awhile that she loves me.

The next day my fever finally broke. We went for a walk to the lake and back. After snacking a bit, I realized that where my fever had left, my libido came back. Upstairs, Erika went down on me in various positions for probably 15 minutes, and I was 90-100% the whole time. It's like a switch got flipped, and it felt amazing. We could do something else for awhile and I'd get softer, but as soon as the attention was back on me I was ready again. I still didn't get close to orgasm, so maybe I've moved up the ladder from PIED to DE, but that's such a huge improvement that I'm not even disappointed.

20 minutes later, she had to get ready to leave and go to work. When she stood up to begin dressing, I embraced her. I got hard immediately and 90% of rational thought drowned just as fast. We haven't had sex yet. Neither of us is in a rush as she's a virgin and I want to wait until I feel like my reboot is over. Well, all I wanted to do was toss her onto the bed and take her, even though we had no form of birth control there. I've always read about men who lose all reason when faced with sex, but I always thought that they were exaggerating since I'd never felt like I would lose control (dopamine desensitization, anyone?). Anyway, I realize now that it's true. I didn't lose control and we didn't have sex, but I know now how powerful that urge can be.

Day 72 — Mood: 8/10 — Libido: 8/10

For the first time in my life, I had full, successful sex!

I put on a condom at first, but that brought me down to 80% so I took it off, deciding I wasn't ready. A bit later, though, it just sort of started happening (without a condom). We went for awhile, then she wanted to stop before there were any "accidents" (though I knew I wasn't close). Afterwards, she used her hands and mouth, and I had my first orgasm in over 70 days. I don't know if you guys get this, but for a couple of minutes before actually coming I was having a miniature orgasm, in which I spasm but don't ejaculate. Then, of course, it felt even better when I was actually ejaculating, and there was a lot.

I feel good about this. I'm glad it happened, but I'd like to learn how to use condoms from now on. Even though it won't be as good, I don't want to start to rely on pulling out. Also, having an orgasm was great, but I don't think I need/want to have one very often. I've really enjoyed being abstinent from orgasm, and I know I can still really enjoy playing around without reaching climax; I haven't even been getting blue balls lately.

Day 72 marks a huge step forward in my journey. My sensitivity has definitely increased from a long time without M or O, and I only expect it to keep getting better. Stay strong, brothers.

Day 79 — Mood: 6/10 — Libido: N/A

So I still have trouble having sex with a condom. I'm not sure at this point how much of my difficulty is physiological and how much is leftover anxiety from many failed attempts at sex, especially when it comes time for putting the condom on. I definitely still associate sex with failure and shame, and when those thoughts come into my head it's difficult to stay in the mood. On the other hand, I am usually hard when playing around clothed, when the possibility of sex isn't in my mind. Well, the only thing to do is practice :)

The last couple of days I was slipping back into using TV and video games as an escape, but like PMO these activities usually leave me feeling worse afterwards, feeling like I'm putting of my life and failing to pursue the missions I really care about. Today was much better. I just have to keep reminding myself of what I *really* want and of what I have to do to achieve those goals. I find it's much more effective to focus on the positive—the things I want and how to make them happen—rather than to preoccupy myself thinking about the things I don't want and how to avoid them.

Day 87 — Mood: 8/10 — Libido: 9/10

Successful sex with a condom! I didn't O, but we went after it for about 20 minutes with next to no PIED problems, and it felt good. The reboot has helped so much, but a big part of recovery for me is also due to being open about my emotions and sexual history/hang-ups with Erika. The weight of unspoken words definitely has a negative effect on my libido, and it is a relief to finally let all of that go. God, it feels so good to finally be getting past this—and to do so with someone I love.

Other areas of my life are going well too. It's like my discipline and motivation from no-PMO has started to carry over into other aspects of my life: I'm getting a good handle on my long-held procrastination habits and other dependencies that hold me back from being who I want to be and doing what I want to do. 2014 is my year, and I'm not wasting it!

Day 94 — Mood: 8/10 — Libido: N/A

So I told my parents all about this. As I said back in my original story, there was never an open dialogue about sex between my parents and their children, so this was definitely a different conversation than we've ever had before. It went well. We all learned a lot, and I think we'll have a more open relationship now. I told them that I will no longer live in ways that make me feel I have to hide parts of my life from my loved ones, and they respected that. I also showed them Gary Wilson's TED talk so they would understand a bit better. I don't think they believed it all, but that's understandable: before I undertook this journey, I didn't really believe it all either.

Also, I said back in my original entry that my parents "seemed utterly sexless" when I was growing up, but it turns out that their relationship isn't what I thought it was—they just kept that part of their lives well segregated from their children.

Day 108 — Mood: 7/10 — Libido: 8/10

Life is good. The ED only shows up occasionally anymore, and it's only when I'm tired or already had sex. During sex I will sometimes lose an erection, but before too long it's back up, and for the most part sex gets better and better each time. I still have severe DE, however. I've had sex (vaginal, oral, manual) quite a few times this last month, and I haven't climaxed a single time. I've only been even a little bit close once or twice. I'm still very much enjoying myself and I don't even get blue balls anymore, but it'd be nice to orgasm once in awhile.

I never had trouble reaching orgasm by myself, but that's probably why it's so difficult to do so without my own hand. I conditioned myself hundreds of times to orgasm from only a certain stimulus, and I'm sure it will take awhile to readjust. Condoms and being circumcised are also factors, however, as they reduce my sensitivity. But I don't feel the need to force it—it will happen when it happens (I hope). Any other guys have a similar experience or words of wisdom?

Day 121 — Mood: 6/10 — Libido: N/A

So I was linked to a random entertainment video off of Facebook today, and from there I followed a link to a page featuring pictures of a certain model—nothing nude or pornographic but certainly enough to get my dopamine surge going. I was captivated, but after scrolling through her pictures for awhile, I realized that the predominant emotion I was feeling was anger.

Awhile ago I read a review of some studies that had been done on the brain. The researchers hooked up electrodes to the limbic systems of rats and allowed the rats to stimulate this area of their brains themselves by pushing a button. They kept pushing that button thousands of times per hour until they collapsed from exhaustion or died from starvation, ignoring food, water, and sexual opportunities. Even when they had to cross electrified flooring in order to push that button, they did it over and over again until their feet were too charred and crippled for them to move. What pleasure these rats must be feeling in order for them to endure such torture, the researchers reasoned. They thought they had found the pleasure centers of the brain.

Further researchers implanted electrodes in human brains as well, and the effect was the same: an almost uncontrollable desire to push the button and self-stimulate. But these subjects reported that it wasn't quite pleasure and satisfaction that they were experiencing—it was a feeling of being on the *brink* of satisfaction, and it was the powerful motivation to reach that satisfaction that kept them pushing the button. But they could never arrive at that feeling of contentment, reporting great frustration with this fact even while wanting to continue. This is because the part of the brain being stimulated was not actually a hub of pleasure but of desire and motivation.

This is how I felt looking at those pictures today. It was like someone was dangling a treat in front of my face, and every time I would reach for it, it would dance a little farther away. And I realized that I **HATE** this feeling. People today use sexually exciting imagery to sell products, collect advertising revenue, or just to satisfy their own egos with "likes" and attention from strangers on the Internet. They know that by activating our desire they can keep us clicking. They know that some of us will associate their products with our desires and pay money to keep pushing the button. They know that even those people they can't fool into opening their wallets will return again and again hoping to acquire satisfaction, upping page views and increasing advertisement revenue. But satisfaction is not what's on offer—only desire. We just end up lost in our own rat cage, pushing a button as slaves to other people's agendas. Those women we see on the Internet are not part of our lives, and they have nothing real to offer us.

I don't count what happened as a relapse because it wasn't porn and I wasn't even tempted to MO, but it wasn't anything good either. Nevertheless I am glad it happened because it taught me something important: I am a pacified button-pushing slave no more. I know where satisfaction is, and it is not to be found in lusting after phantoms on a computer screen. That's no longer me. Now, I see what I want in the real world and I take it, and life is beautiful.

Day 136 — Mood: 7/10 — Libido: N/A

I saw an interview with an ex-porn actress the other day. She told some hard truths about the industry, detailing the manipulative, uncaring way it treats the young women it recruits. Most use alcohol or drugs to numb themselves in order to get through shooting a scene, and they often suffer vaginal, anal, and throat tears, infections, and other abuse. I can't do her story justice.

I know that some women in porn say that they enjoy their work, that it empowers them sexually. I know these women are out there (though some may be paid to say these things), but many, many of them are vulnerable individuals predated upon by men wanting to exploit them for money and sexual gratification. When I used porn, I didn't really care about this.

I'm reminded of before I was a vegan. Even then I knew that factory farms produced most of our animal products—places where animals are subjected to painful, joyless lives until they are violently killed. But there were also some animals that were raised with some concern for humane treatment, so I just assumed that the animal products I ate came from these creatures. I pretended, embracing ignorance for my own comfort. Five years ago I stopped eating animals for my own health, but through that journey I also realized that I didn't want any part in their mistreatment. Five months ago I stopped using porn for my own health, and now I realize that I don't want any part in the mistreatment of people, either.

Day 138 — Mood: 8/10 — Libido: 9/10

For awhile I got a bit complacent in this journey. I would indulge in fantasy, especially when waking up. I would rub myself a bit for a couple of minutes but not even approach orgasm, so I didn't count it as edging. I also started to click on some sexual—though not explicit— links and get turned on by these false stimuli. I knew I wasn't going to masturbate to these things; it was more about satisfying a curiosity than anything else. Then a couple of weeks ago I realized that I was slipping down a dangerous path and also felt that my progress with DE was stalling. I needed to change something, so I went back to how I started this journey: no fantasy, no self-touching, no pixels that turn me on. And it is so much easier this way. No longer do I have to struggle with myself to decide whether or not to pursue some borderline material: I just don't do it.

Even better, today I had an orgasm just from sex with a condom— twice. Not only has my PIED disappeared, but my DE seems to be on the way out as well! I think the sudden improvement was due in part to the return of my zero-tolerance policy and in part because of some new positions we tried that worked better for my orgasm. It took almost five months to get here, but this process absolutely works. I not only fixed my sexual dysfunction as I set out to do: I also accepted and shared myself with those close to me, grew in willpower, motivation, and maturity, and I found love. Thanks again to everyone who has shared their stories. I now consider my own story a complete success.

Day 150 — Mood: All over the place — Libido: N/A

So I got dumped today. It was very surprising. Though I had a bad feeling about our relationship for the last few days, she never talked to me about any issues and now refuses to see me after breaking it off over the phone. At first I was shocked, then sad, then confused and angry. I immediately hopped on my motorcycle and went to see my best friend, and we spent the next several hours wandering around the city talking and meeting new people.

I could write all sorts of conjecture about what I think is going on in her head, but I really don't know, so I'll just write about me. I really loved her, but I lost a lot of respect for her today when she didn't have the guts to talk to me in person and try to come to a mutual understanding. It probably wouldn't have saved our relationship, but it would have given us a chance at separating amicably with a sense of closure. Our memories together feel like smoke—like a dream—and I'm left with the cold sound of her voice on my cell phone.

But it wasn't a dream, and I grew a lot these last five months we were together. Most importantly, I was faithful to myself and have no regrets about my choices. I wish we could have had that closure, but I realize that just because a story doesn't have a satisfying ending doesn't mean it wasn't a good story.

As for porn, a lot of guys relapse after a breakup, and it did occur to me. But half of a moment later the thought of giving her the power to send me down so low almost made me vomit. I will not be relapsing.

I have to admit that there was a small part of me that was relieved after she broke us off. I could see myself spending a long time with this woman, and the thought of being with one woman—even her—for potentially the rest of my life did scare me. I wasn't sure how I was going to reconcile my desire to be with her with my desire to be free. Thanks to her that conflict is now over. That small glad part of me has kept growing and growing over the last several hours to become a powerful optimism and excitement for all the possibility of the world, and right now I feel charged with life. I'm sure I'll be going up and down emotionally over the following days, but I am such a stronger and better man than I was six months ago, and that thought fills me with joy.

Johnny's in his room again (parenting: porn and sex)

Technology has become a central hub of the modern world, dominating our lives at work, at home, and at play, and none are more susceptible to the temptations of entertainment technology than children. In America, 8-18 year-olds average seven hours and 38 minutes of entertainment media use each day.[58] That is half of their waking lives. 83% of all American households have an Internet connection,[59] which provides our children with unprecedented access to an unlimited supply of information. And they will use it. When they need to write a paper about Thomas Jefferson, they use the Internet. When they want to play a video game or find movie show times, they use the Internet. When they are turned on or confused about sex, they use the Internet. All it takes to pursue almost any curiosity is a Google search, and all children become curious about sex. And, unfortunately, as much good information about sex as there is on the Internet, there is much more hardcore porn.

Many adults are uncomfortable talking about sex with their children—or even with their friends or spouses. If you are one of these people, get over it. We can no longer afford to avoid the topic of sex or delay it until our children's teenage years. Decades ago children may have been able to find their own way to a healthy romantic life, but home Internet access has changed that. No longer are young persons figuring it out for themselves: instead, the Internet is their teacher, and it has just as much or more potential to teach unhealthy promiscuity, objectification, and addiction as it has to teach healthy sex practices. Sex education has become a race between the Internet and you, the parent. If you are the first one to provide your child with honest, complete information about sex, love, and porn, then your child will be armed with a solid foundation of knowledge with which to confront the very warped, confusing world he or she will undoubtedly be exposed to, whether online or off.

---

[58] Generation M2: Media in the lives of 8- to 18-year-olds. (2010, January). *Kaiser Family Foundation*. Web.

[59] Over three-quarters of U.S. households get broadband at home. (2013, September 26). *Leichtman Research Group | Press Releases*. Web.

Neither can parents rely on schools' sex education classes to teach their children everything they need to know. Most of these classes are woefully inadequate or come too late, but even the best sex education classes do not replace open communication between parent and child. Children respect and love their parents, and children will trust their parents' word as long as it is honest and forthright. Our children need a home environment in which they are comfortable discussing sex. When parents provide that environment, their children will come to them for answers. If the subject of sex seems at all taboo, uncomfortable, or shameful, then children will seek answers elsewhere and shove sex into the "never talk about with parents" shoebox, right beside drug use and their dreams of skipping college to become a street magician. The answers and sexual outlets that children find among their friends and online are more likely to be harmful than helpful, and you will have missed a chance at a fully open and honest relationship with your children.

The first step toward avoiding this trap is to educate yourself about sex. It is more likely than not that your own sex education was inadequate, so fix it. The Internet is a phenomenal source of information as long as you can differentiate the trustworthy sources from the untrustworthy ones. Find out who wrote what you read on the Internet, and decide for yourself if they have the authority to educate you about sex. Learn everything you can, and get comfortable discussing sex with your friends and/or spouse. Children are very receptive, so if you project reluctance or discomfort they will pick up on it and try to eject from an awkward conversation—which is why you must first practice with other adults.

Dismiss the idea that there is one "sex talk" that parents have with their children before putting the topic to bed. Sex is a very important part of life, so it should be a common topic of discussion throughout your children's lives. Sex education begins early. It is common for very young children to ask questions about gender and genitals and to explore their own bodies and masturbate. They may be too young to process everything about sex, so do not overload them with information on your first conversation. However, it is very important at this time of children's development to answer their questions honestly and satisfy their curiosity with the truth. Do not gloss over the real information with euphemisms, put off answering their questions until they are older, or rush through the conversation. Use correct language, such as "penis" and "vagina", and take your time. Answer their questions completely, make sure they understand by asking them to explain the information back to you, and finish the conversation by asking if they have any more questions and assuring them that if they think of any more then they can always come to you.

If your young child is touching him- or herself or masturbating, do not snap in anger, try to distract him or her, or avoid the topic. Doing any of these things only communicates that sexual pleasure is shameful and not to be talked about, which is an attitude that can last a lifetime. Instead, say that what he or she is doing is called "masturbation", and most people do it at some time or another. It is important, though, to not do it in public because it makes some people uncomfortable, so save it for private time.

As your children get older, maintain this forthright attitude. If they ask you something that you are not sure about, just admit that you do not know and suggest that you research the answer together. This will allow you an opportunity to demonstrate how good research is done (on sex or any other topic). Show them some websites or other sources that you trust for good information and explain why you trust them. If you come across some suspect information, explain how they can tell that this author might not know what he or she is talking about, and stress that it is always good to check multiple sources and then discuss with you what they find so that you can discover the right answers together.

As far as encouraging abstinence versus safe sex, I do not presume to dictate what moral views you try to instill in your children, but I can recommend that you are more likely to succeed in fostering a healthy adult if you explain the reasons for your beliefs and open up an honest, comprehensive dialogue rather than just enforcing rules. A recent federal survey studying four abstinence-only sex education programs showed that they resulted in "no impacts on rates of sexual abstinence" and "no differences in rates of unprotected sex."[60]

On the other hand, a University of Washington review of national survey data showed that those who received comprehensive sex education were the least likely to engage in intercourse and 60% less likely than those who received no sex education and 50% less likely than those who received abstinence-only education to get pregnant or

---

[60] Trenholm, C., Devaney, B., Fortson, K., Quay, L., Wheeler, J., & Clark, M. (2007, April 1). Impacts of four Title V, Section 510 abstinence education programs . *Mathematica Policy Research*. Web.

impregnate someone during teen years. Mississippi, the state with the highest rate of teen pregnancy, does not require sex education, but when it is given, abstinence-only education is the state standard. Conversely, the state with the lowest rate of teen pregnancy, New Hampshire, requires comprehensive sex education in schools, which includes information about abstinence, condoms, and contraception.[61]

The message here is clear and unsurprising: Knowledge leads to smart decisions; ignorance leads to mistakes. Wanting to protect your children from the world is natural, but the truth is that they live in this world and need correct knowledge in order to navigate it. Whatever beliefs you would like to pass on, trying to keep your children in the dark is not an effective way to encourage moral or intelligent behavior.

As for discussing pornography, the correct time to broach the subject is not after you discover some disturbing web history on the family computer, as this is likely to feel more like a confrontation. Instead, bring it up as soon as your child starts using the Internet. If you have already created an easygoing dialogue about sex, then talking about porn will not be difficult. If you have read this book thus far, then you are qualified to teach your children all they need to know about Internet porn. Tell them that there are websites on the Internet on which people upload sexual pictures, videos, and stories and that this is called "pornography" or "porn" for short. Tell them that many people enjoy looking at these things and masturbating to them, but that you have learned how harmful this habit can become. Tell them that porn takes the love out of sex, and tell them how porn use can disrupt their natural sexual development and lead to relationship and sexual problems in the future. If they ask for details about these problems, share those details. Tell them that you know it is natural to be curious but that it is better to wait and satisfy that curiosity in real life with a loving partner, and tell them that you do not want porn in your house.

Logistically, there are several steps you can take to foster healthy Internet use in your family. You should not allow children to have personal computers in their rooms; there is no reason to invite temptation, no matter how responsible your children are. Instead, keep a family computer in a common area in which it is easy for anyone to see the screen, making it clear that privacy is not something to be expected while on the computer. Installing ad-blocking and Internet

---

[61] Beadle, A. (2012, April 10). Teen pregnancies highest in states with abstinence-only policies. *ThinkProgress*. Web.

filter software can be helpful in preventing accidental viewing of adult content, but this software cannot wholly block a determined attempt to get around it. Internet accountability software, on the other hand, simply tracks web use and sends reports to your email, allowing you to keep an account of Internet use in your home and open a discussion with your family if you see anything inappropriate. Recommended software can be found in the "Additional resources" section. If your Internet Service Provider provides a proprietary adult-content filter, ask them to activate it.

If you do discover that your child is using porn, whether online or off, it is very important to maintain a calm and easygoing dialogue rather than confronting your child with anger and disappointment. Say that you understand how tempting it can be to use porn to satisfy sexual curiosity, and there is no reason to dole out punishment for natural desires. But porn is an unhealthy expression of those natural desires that can lead to very real sexual and emotional consequences, jeopardizing future relationships and happiness for momentary pleasure. Share this book with them. Also know that like adults adolescents often use porn to fill absences in their lives. If they feel unfulfilled, unmotivated, or socially insecure, porn can provide an addictive temporary relief. Take it as a sign that your child may need more of your time and attention in positive ways. Have fun or learn new skills together, ask about your child's interests, and encourage those passions. Try to help find more social clubs or group activities for him or her to participate in with others of a similar age.

If you have already created a sex-negative atmosphere in your household and regret it, you are not too late to forge a more honest and open relationship with your children. Think long and hard about how your own parents handled discussions about sex, whether that was healthy or not, how you have discussed sex with your own children, and how you would like to change. If you feel like you have wronged your children with your old attitudes and behaviors, then start the conversation with them by apologizing. Tell them that you have been doing a lot of thinking and decided that you want to change how your family talks about sex. Tell them how your own parents talked to you about sex and how that influenced your life and your parenting style. Tell them what you regret as a parent and why, as well as how you would like to change. Tell them that you are tired of avoiding topics like sex and want to be comfortable talking about anything with them. Tell them that whatever your mistakes in the past, now you only want to help them and support them, not judge or punish them for their choices. Ask them how they feel about all this and if they have any suggestions.

Depending on how old they are and your family's history with sex, shame, etc., your children may already be firmly uncomfortable discussing certain parts of their lives with you and will resist open communication. Do not be discouraged. It will simply take time for them to believe that they are safe talking to you and that they will not be judged, shamed, or punished for being honest (so do not judge, shame, or punish them when they do open up). Do not pressure your children to talk to you about their own private lives as this will only cause them to retreat further into their shells. Instead, make sex, drugs, and other taboo topics a more common feature of family conversation. Bring up something you learned, such as a fact about childbirth or conception that you find interesting, and ask your children if they knew about it. Did they learn that in sex education class? As your children become used to this safer environment for communication, they will naturally start to open up, ask questions, and volunteer information—but they will only do this if they do not feel threatened or pushed.

One of the most powerful techniques for helping your child to relax and open up is to share your own story. Tell them about your own embarrassing or shameful history with sex, masturbation, porn, alcoholism, gambling, excessive gum chewing, etc. and how you conquered your demons. Famed psychologist Carl Jung wrote, "The most important gift a parent can give a child is to tell them about their dark side. Telling children about your struggles helps them developmentally to have a realistic picture of what it means to be human."[62] Teens can feel too intimidated to be honest with parents who seem perfect—and therefore unable to empathize with and understand a teen who is making mistakes and feels inadequate in comparison. Show them that you, too, are fallible and vulnerable to temptation, and also that vices can be overcome. Your example of trust and honesty is likely to inspire them to do the same, though not necessarily right away. This technique may seem scary, but how can you expect your children to feel comfortable being honest with you if you cannot lead by example and be honest with them? On the other hand, do not burden and confuse children too young with your baggage.

---

[62] Black, C., Dillon, D., Carnes, S. (2003). Disclosure to children: Hearing the child's experience. *Sexual addiction & Compulsivity*, 10(1).

Teenagers are usually ready to hear about their parents' flaws, but each child's needs and capacities are individual and must be assessed by you, the parent.

The above technique works well when discussing struggles that you have overcome, as resolved history poses little threat to your children's sense of security. When your struggle (with porn addiction or any other compulsive behavior) is current, however, disclosure to your children can still be beneficial but must be facilitated with greater care. Mishandled disclosure or sharing with children too young may confuse them, compromise their faith in family unity, or burden them with the responsibility to choose sides or provide emotional support to one or both parents. On the other hand, an atmosphere of secrets and shame in the home can also be oppressive and confusing to children, many of whom may handle the stress better if they could discuss why their parents are arguing and what is being done to fix the situation.

Often, parents far overestimate how well a secret addiction has been kept from their children. In a survey of children of sex addicts, "Sixty of eighty-nine respondents indicated they knew of their parent's behavior prior to disclosure."[63] Though many of these children did not know the full extent of the addiction, they knew or suspected parts of it. This partial knowledge can engender doubt and insecurity; they come to yearn for an open discussion and reassurance that the family will get better and stay together—or at least that none of this is the children's fault and that both parents will always love them.

The degree of disclosure that is appropriate depends on the children's age and maturity as well as the nature of the issue, though disclosure should always be a united effort by both parents whenever possible. In cases of current sexual addiction in one or both parents, experts suggest disclosing the full nature of the problem no earlier than mid-adolescence, except where the child needs the information for his or her own safety or is in danger of hearing about the problem from another source. Younger children, however, can still be told about their parents' marital and personal problems in more general terms, along with reassurance that the parents are working hard to solve the issue. Before talking to your child about a parent's current addiction, see "Disclosure to Children: Hearing the Child's Experience" in the "Additional resources" section for a more complete guide to disclosure.

---

[63] Black, C., Dillon, D., Carnes, S. (2003). Disclosure to children: Hearing the child's experience. *Sexual addiction & Compulsivity*, 10(1).

No one can guarantee that our children will not get pregnant too young, become porn addicts, contract an STD, defy our values, or internalize our own struggles with addiction. The best we can do is to create a genuinely honest, loving, and trusting family dynamic. So let's go do our best.

Final Words

Several authors have referenced a certain Native American legend in relation to recovering from porn addiction. In this legend, a grandfather counsels his grandson, who is struggling with destructive impulses. The grandfather says, "Inside every human being a constant battle rages, a battle between two wolves. One is evil—he is full of hate, lust, greed, and arrogance. The other wolf is good—full of love, compassion, honesty, and humility. These two wolves are constantly at war, both trying to dominate the individual." The grandson considers this for a moment, then asks, "Which wolf will win?" His grandfather replies, "Whichever one you feed."

This story is supposed to demonstrate that the desires you choose to feed become strong, while the desires you starve die out; thus you may shape your habits and your life. This fact is absolutely true. However, I have heard a different version of the story.

In this other version, the grandfather has a bit more to say. When the boy asks, "Which wolf will win?" the grandfather responds, "If you feed them right, then they both win. Understand, if I starve the dark wolf then he becomes desperate for my attention and jealous of his brother, biting my heels at every turn and constantly fighting the white wolf, whom I feed well. I will never know peace because I am torn inside from denying a part of myself. But if I feed the dark wolf, then he is happy and the white wolf is happy and they work together to serve me. You see, the dark wolf has many fine qualities—ambition, tenacity, courage, ferocity, and cunning—that I need sometimes and that the white wolf cannot give me. But the white wolf has empathy, strength, compassion, and a communal spirit.

"In the end, the white wolf needs his brother by his side—not at his throat. To feed only one wolf means to starve the other, and then you are at war with yourself. To care well for both wolves means that they will follow you faithfully and use their strengths for nothing that is not a part of your great purpose. Feed them both and you will be at peace inside. And when you have peace, you can listen to those voices of deep knowledge that guide you truly in every choice. Peace is our mission, grandson. A man at peace has greatness inside of him. A man at war with himself has nothing."

WACK

Addicted to Internet Porn
By Noah B.E. Church

whack off (wăk ŏf) *Slang*
v.intr
To masturbate.

+

porn

=

wack (wăk) *Slang*
adj. **wack·er**, **wack·est**
Very bad.

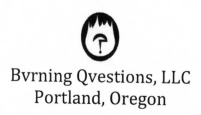

Bvrning Qvestions, LLC
Portland, Oregon

Testimonies, success stories, and advice

Thousands of men and women have shared publicly their stories of how porn use has affected their lives. In the following pages are the accounts and advice of just a small percentage of them. I have tried to compile as many different perspectives as possible by including statements from the young and the old, men and women, porn addicts and partners of porn addicts, casual users and hard cases. I hope that from their failures and successes you may draw inspiration and wisdom. Read straight through or refer to the following table to find those most interesting to you.

Anonymous:

To be honest, when I first learned all about porn addiction I lowered my head into my hands and wept—not because of all the years I realized I had wasted, but because I now had hope of beating this demon that had possessed me for decades.

"Saved my marriage and maybe even my life"

John: Hello my fellow rebooters.

I am officially calling my reboot a success. After 90 days of no PMO I have successfully realigned my brain, broken my porn addiction, and had the most amazing sex of my life. This reboot has done so much more for me than fixing my penis, it has saved my marriage and maybe even my life.

For a detailed version of my back story you can read it in my journal.

The short version: I had been addicted to hardcore/extreme pornography since age 16 (I am 28 now). The addiction has given me minor ED, inability to O during any sexual encounter that is not my hand, decreased my libido, and stolen a lot of my manliness.

When my wife found my porn collection it almost cost me my marriage, she left me taking our baby daughter away, and I went into a depressed mental breakdown with suicidal thoughts. My life got back on track when my wife sent me a link to "www.yourbrainonporn.com".

So after 90 days of no PMO (with more than a little support from this amazing forum), my wife and I are very strong together. She understands my addiction and is very supportive. We have started having sex again and it is far better than sex used to be. I have so much more desire for her now. I want to be intimate with her and not sit in the dark with my computer. My brain feels healthier, I can think clearer, I have less anxiety (although I do still have some, but that's other issues). There was so much in my life that I wrote off as me being weird, that I never knew it was wrong or broken in the first place. But it seems that each day I am finding something new that porn has taken away from me but that my reboot has given back.

With my reboot I went complete. No orgasms including sex, no exposure to sexual images or material (looking away or avoiding all movies that contained any nudity/sexual content), no fantasizing, no checking out chicks on the street, no touching my penis in any sexual way.

111

So my secrets to success...THE RIGHT HEADSPACE.

The classic "mistake" that I see from other rebooters is that they miss masturbation or porn. They think that they have to deny themselves this awesome feeling that you get when you masturbate.

Going 90+ days without any sexual release is hard for normal people. For us porn addicts it's even harder. During reboot you will be in pain, your balls will hurt, you will get mood swings, depression. You will get massive cravings for porn and masturbation. You are literally trying to change the chemicals in your brain. Your brain will try and trick you into looking or doing something you shouldn't because it is being starved of dopamine. If you in any way think of masturbation or porn as something you miss, you will break.

Porn and masturbation destroyed your manhood. Why would you miss the thing that has given you ED, or anxiety, or whatever reason it is why you are here. You need to want to give it up, but more than that you need to not look upon masturbation as a good thing. Don't fall for your brain telling you to test your penis because you've been in flatline for a while. That's your porn starved brain playing tricks on you! Your penis will be fine. It's not going to break because you haven't touched it, it's going to get better. Every day that goes past that you don't touch your penis is another day closer to you being better.

Rebooting is hard, but I never questioned it. I never wanted to give up. I felt the urge to watch porn, or masturbate, but I never even thought about giving in because I didn't just want to give up porn, I needed to. If I didn't then I would have lost my family, and I would go through anything to keep my family. I needed to get off porn as much as I needed to breathe, and I am successful.

And my quest isn't over. I am going a lifetime without porn and like an alcoholic I will need to be vigilant.

Hello, my name is John and I am a porn addict. I have been off PMO for 91 days now and I have never felt better. I would like to tell you all that you can do it. You can change your brain. All you need is the right headspace and you can do anything.

My friends you are not alone in this, and if anyone would like my help, support, or advice I will be here.

Update: Hey guys just wanted to post an update. It's been a while since I've been on here but things have been going great. I've come such a long way since giving up PMO.

So the big news is that I have made my wife pregnant again—this time naturally. As in from having regular sex. This is our second baby, and the first time she got pregnant was when I was on PMO and I could never O from sex so had to finish by hand…every time. Now I always O with sex and the sex is sooooooo much better. It seems strange to me now that I could just always tell myself that it was just me being a bit strange that meant I could not O, boy was I wrong.

Giving up PMO has made such a big difference in my life. It really has saved my marriage. Good luck to you all. I hope you have as much success as I have had.

Update: So I'm coming up on a full year of no PMO. Feels good to have made it this far. I'm still only having O through sex which is fantastic. Sex is still so much better than it ever used to be before the reboot.

I have been contemplating the changes in my life since I have gone on the no PMO journey. Last night after my wife went to bed I did some cleaning in the kitchen and framed a piece of art that I have had for over 2 years just sitting in a cupboard. This is stuff I never would have done before as I would have just snuck off to PMO. I got so much fulfillment by framing the art piece and in a strange way it's something I only have done because of giving up porn. Instead of damaging my brain I am using my time to improve my house and surroundings. It feels really good to have the time to do that instead of feeling compulsions to go off and PMO at every available opportunity. It's a small thing but a big change to me.

Good luck on your journey my friends, and remember to appreciate all the victories of the journey, even the little things.

"If you're struggling, keep struggling"

Constantin: I've been meaning to write this up for a while. I am no longer subscribed to NoFap so it slipped my mind. I unsubscribed not because I gave up but because I no longer need support to not fap.

I've still wandered to porn sites now and again but after clicking on the first video I just feel kind of dumb and close it within a minute or so.

I was never terribly addicted but did NoFap more as a test. I still feel much more in control and overall happier. I talk to girls A LOT and I barely need to "spit game". I get looks and just ask for their contact info and it's basically pretty easy. Sure I still get rejected but it doesn't faze me, because I have no idea where she is at in life. Maybe her cat just died, maybe she has a boyfriend that she's very happy with or maybe she just hates guys with facial hair. Who knows?

Since starting, I've been training for the Beijing marathon which I will compete in in about two weeks, and I'm gonna kick its ass.

I just got back from Bali this past week after fulfilling my 10-year dream of learning to surf and while I was there met an incredible Korean girl that I had a short fling with.

Not to say that every part of my life is great now, but it's much easier to see the parts that need focus and a lot of my old bullshit has fallen away to reveal the core of importance in my life.

As for superpowers...well the above is "super" enough for me. Being able to feel my emotions more fully—both happiness and sadness—is a great gift.

If you're struggling, keep struggling. Life is about challenging and leaving behind the weaker versions of yourself. Don't give up. Ever. You won't regret it.

Apeman:

I'm feeling on top of the world lately. I'm comfortable with the idea of never watching porn again. That idea always made me a little anxious before, but now I know that the real world is more satisfying than an infinite porn harem.

And we choose one or the other.

"I am happy"

Anonymous: Within a week after ridding my life of porn and masturbation, I started to feel an entirely new sensation, a warm ache that started in my gut and extended all the way to the tip of my penis. Not long after, my wife and I had the most exciting sex of our lives. I am nearly 60.

Since then this new need for my wife has only increased, and neither fantasy nor porn are able to distract me. My desire is only fulfilled with her now, and we are trying to make up for all of the years in which I wasn't fit to experience true intimacy with her. Do I regret those years? Yes. But even more than regret I feel so, so glad that I found YBOP and the stories of so many other men. I owe you all my life.

For those of you who are where I was, please just listen to my story. I have made a lot of mistakes—affairs, lies, more and more extreme porn—but even at my age I was able to change my life, and I am so grateful that I did. It has been four months since I last PMO'd, and I do still think about going back to it when things get difficult, but I'm taking it one day at a time. Honestly, I delayed addressing my issues for so long that I'm not sure if I'll ever fully heal all of the scars. My one saving grace was that I didn't have the Internet when I was young. Looking back, there is a huge difference between the porn of my youth and high-speed Internet porn. Multiple windows, multiple tabs, all with different women and ever more extreme porn—the dopamine rush is on an entirely different level. It took only a couple of years of this before my energy and motivation started to crash. I was depressed, I was unhappy with my life. I even considered killing myself.

But four months into this new life, I am happy. Don't get me wrong, I still have a lot of problems, but I have my wife, and I feel myself come to life just holding her in my arms.

Anonymous:

This addiction is powerful, possibly the greatest challenge I have ever faced, and I'm not sure how to proceed and haven't found the time to look into it because, well, I've been jacking off too much. I'm trapped in my own little porn world, and when I'm there I'm pretty damn content riding wave after wave of endorphin goodness.

So here I am. I say content, but that's not true. Inside I know this is an endeavor that I should not abandon. But I'm not sure how to restart. I turn 40 this weekend. My goal had been to kick this before that and I sure thought I would. But the willpower isn't there and the pull for PMO is, and it's strong as a mother fucker.

"Doing Hard Things"

LampitosGames: Wow. 3 months already? I find it a little bit hard to believe myself that I made it this far. I woke up one day and decided I would never fap again, that is simply it. That day was 3 years ago, lol. I've woken up with that same idea countless times in my head, and I cannot count the number of times I proved myself wrong. About 91 days ago, I found this sub-reddit. For the longest time, I was trying to quit for religious reasons, and I had no idea what kind of real benefits this NoFap thing could provide. Once I saw YBOP, and all the videos over there, I was all in. That was the tipping point of the iceberg. Something went off in my head, and I realized how much of a mess I was in. I put things off until the night before, I was never motivated to

115

do anything except sit down and play games, I was in terrible physical condition (and arguably mental condition as well). I had goals, but I pushed them into tomorrow and told myself I have time, I'm only fifteen.

People nowadays, at least the ones I know, are afraid of *Doing Hard Things*. That is the simple truth that our society is built around, the American lifestyle of please yourself as much as you want whenever you want no matter if it costs others much more than your comfort is worth. That is not what anybody wants to be, but somehow 99% of society fits the description of average. School, too! The question I hear most often is "Will this be on the test?" and not "Why does that work?". Some wire or neuron broke in my head that day. It was the catalyst for a chain reaction that has flipped my world-view on its head. I know most of this does not seem relevant, but you will put it all together soon enough. I might not be the best in the world at maths or programming, but I am "so good *for my age*", as everyone likes to put it. I was often tempted to be content with my 'prodigy' status. I could get A's and B's without studying for a single test all year, and it only piled on more of my "I'm better than everyone else" attitude. I do not know what snapped me out of floating by without trying, but something did. I assume it was a combination of my poor physical condition, worsening depression & social anxiety, and loneliness (Oddly, the day before I began NoFap, I was having a little pity-party because it marked 1 year without a relationship. "I, like God, do not play with dice and do not believe in coincidence" -V for Vendetta). So, mindlessly browsing the Internet like a zombie looking for more porn to shovel onto the pile, I found myself here. I was not cynical of this reddit, quite the contrary. I was surprised that people other than me were trying to stop fapping. No more than 10 minutes into my browsing, I found /r/getmotivated as well. I stayed up well into the night, and instead of fapping I flooded every part of my brain with people overcoming the (what others say) impossible. I sat down, looked at my life, and decided I was not the person I wanted to be.

I cannot really explain how this all happened so quickly. I have learned a lot in the past three months, arguably more than I have learned in my entire life. If I want to become the elite, I have to start now, while all of my competitors are fapping their lives away. Every nerd ever plays games and says "Man, I wish I could make something this awesome!". I had the same mindset, I *wanted* to program cool games, I even had a ton of ideas; but like everything else, I pushed all of that onto my future self. My future self was the guy who had it together in college and was a programming whiz. I was completely depressed, I had social anxiety (clinical, like I had it before I found porn), my face was covered with acne, I had nearly 0 friends. I convinced myself that playing video games 7+ hours on the weekdays and 16+ hours on the weekends was an okay thing to do because I needed experience in games to be able to make them. I actually believed that "I am addicted to video games" would look good on a résumé.

Okay, enough about my back story, that's all good and everything, but it does not really matter. 90 day reports are not the "why I'm here" reports. 90 days is the point where the soldier files a field-report for all his fellow trainees who aren't quite there yet. For those of you wondering, no, I do not have a girlfriend. This is all hardmode! It is possible, and I see no future stopping date either. The "superpowers" are not superpowers, they are all the things fapping has taken away from you. I remember 60 days, and how I was lying in bed crying uncontrollably because all my emotions were flooding back in so quickly I had no idea what was going on. It's like being handed *the force* from star wars, having no training, and then trying to use it. It does not work. At first, your head is just swirling around in a pool, and slowly you learn to control your emotions, and they are stronger than ever! Now, instead of random crazy depression, I get random happy bursts, where I feel like I can do anything at all! If you told me a year ago that I would be working out every day, I would tell you that you had gone insane. Well, here I am. Working out is something that I cannot stress enough, it helps clear your head, fight off urges, and just improves your life in general. My acne is falling off a cliff right now, it is disappearing, disintegrating, whatever you want to say about it. I have thrown procrastination out of the door. I am more motivated to do whatever I set my heart to. My focus has shot through the roof, I had ADD, but now I can sit down and work on homework for hours without a break. My anxiety is not gone, however. That existed before fapping, and probably will be in the back of my head for life. However, I have magically gained the power to beat up the little idiot who tells me I can't talk to women or that I shouldn't go hang out with friends. I'm sure there is more, and I'm sure I would know exactly what it all was if I relapsed today. They say you don't know what you have till it is gone, and I assume I have grown in ways that I don't realize. Dating is something I do not plan to do until possibly next year. I need to focus on the fundamentals of my life, and fine-tune myself into who I want to be before I date. I'm perfectly fine with waiting, though. I can still talk to women, and when I get the chance to do so, I'm quite good at it.

This is a wonderful community, and I always see the question "Any tips for a n00b/person who is new?". My advice to you, friend, is do whatever it takes. First off, commit pornocide, delete your ENTIRE collection. I do not care how attached you are, but if you are serious about NoFap, and you still have it, your logic fails. You are trying to quit your addiction but saving your stash for "later". It is like a recovering alcoholic keeping his cupboard stocked full of his favorite beer 24/7. Next on the list, read the sidebar! Read everything on YBOP. Learn as much as you can. Cram it all into your brain. There is no such thing as "I cannot learn anymore". Trust me, I've tried to learn "too much" in these past three months. It does not work. Look at yourself now, then look at who you would like to be in 10 years. How do you get there? Small, daily steps add up to staggering long-term results. Exercise! Holy crap I cannot say this enough. "I do not have a gym membership" is NEVER an excuse. I haven't been to the gym ever. Like not in my life. Start by doing as many push-ups as you can do (does not matter if it is a low number), then do the same for sit-ups, crunches, planking, leg lifts (all four: back, side, side, front), and bench dips. Okay, you did as many as you can? Good, now, take the lowest number, and the next night, do that many of every exercise. Then, after that, add 1 rep for every single day! Read books, books are good. If you do not know what to read, I suggest "Fahrenheit 451", All the hunger games books, "The Book Thief", The Inheritance Series (Eragon, Eldest, Brisingr, & Inheritance), "Looking for Alaska", and everything Tolkien has ever written. Pursue your hobbies! Limit your facebook/reddit time. And most of all, never give up!

"Thank you"

Anonymous: As a living, breathing, non-porn woman, I can't thank all of you enough for what you're doing.

This generation's excessive use of Internet porn terrifies me. The constant influx of new bodies, new kinks, new faces and breasts and buttocks flashing on screens in an unending search for perfection and an ever-hotter sex object freaks me out beyond belief. I know what a guy does in his alone time isn't my business, but in the end what scares me is this: **I can't compete with that.**

I'm human. I'm one person. I can't be edited or cropped or only shown at my best angle. I have stubble and creases and blemishes and veins, I'm not tanned and oiled and lubed up and prancing around in a thong all day. What I'm finding is that the young men I'm with, even the ones who claim I'm the most beautiful creature they've ever seen (and they do) aren't aroused by just me. I could get completely naked, sit on his lap, put my real hands on him and kiss him with real lips, and I'm still second best. I can't be opened in five tabs as a brunette and a redhead and with huge boobs and small ones and thinner and curvier and the rest. I'm stagnant, stationary, one being. And somehow that's not sexy.

Women NEED NoFappers. We need to be sexy again. We need a guy who can look at his girlfriend, his fiancée, his wife, and find her attractive. I'm looking for that, and I hope I find it, because in the end I can't settle for less. I can't waste my time trying to fix myself and deal with rejection and disappointment because he couldn't stay away from a hundred other, new, sexier girls. It's too heartbreaking.

So thank you, each and every one of you, for doing what you're doing (or not doing, I should say). You're getting back to normal, you're standing up and saying to the world, "Sex should be sexy! Men should want their women more than their computers!" You're giving me hope that I'm good enough, that it's okay for me to be who I am, and that I can have a normal and fulfilling sex life.

If you're ever feeling weak or considering going back to the cycle of binging and craving and self-loathing, stay strong for us girls. You're the Prince Charmings of the 21st century, because if he could have stayed home and pulled up "princessXXX18.com" she'd still be locked in that tower. You're a new breed of heroes, and I hope I can find someone like you to sweep me off my feet and mean it.

Thank you.

I'm a better father because of NoFap

thibaultguy: When I was in the heyday of fapping, I think I was a really bad father. I used to be very irritated with my nine-year-old daughter when she would want to spend some time with me.

Although the primary breadwinner, I work from home and have set up a nice office room there. She would come into my office after school to say "Hi" and spend some time with me, but I would be really irritated though I would do my best not to show it. I would secretly wish for her to go out of the office and leave me alone. I am very certain now that this irritation was due to me wanting to go back to browsing online porn.

After I started no PMO'ing almost 80 days ago, I have not experienced any irritation whatsoever. I have developed a routine of having her sit in my office room and complete her homework as she was not doing too well at school lately. She loves it, and I think she is thriving. I love it because I am lucky enough to spend time with her regularly. Now I miss her when she's not around.

This change was so subtle that I never realized it until I thought about it today while reading a few articles on "yourbrainonporn.com", and then it hit me: I am becoming a better father because I not only have time to help my daughter with her homework, but I also absolutely enjoy spending time with her (like a normal parent should). I've actually increased the time I spend with her and have even started preparing her lunch and sometimes her dinner for her. I even step away from my laptop to go out of my office and eat at the table like a normal person should. Every day I feel so blessed at having been able to take the step to stop something that I had no idea was affecting me in such a negative way.

How NoFap not changed, but saved my life—100 Day Report

K.V.: Okay guys. I didn't really know if I want to write a report or not, but I feel like I owe you one. I want to tell you about myself before NoFap, while doing the 100 days and how I feel now.

Before NoFap—Rock bottom

2011: 5'7, 125 lbs, 19 years old. I was addicted to a lot of stuff. Games, porn, alcohol, weed, amphetamine, LSD, LSA, shrooms, every psychedelic drug basically. They helped me to forget. My mother kicked me out when I was 18 because I "needed to learn to stand on my own feets", so I had to move to a really shitty apartment in a city far from home where I don't know anybody. I got a shitty underpaid 9-to-5 job in a local office making $4/hr with shitty coworkers and a boss who only wants to become rich. It was barely enough to pay the bills. Needless to say I had suicidal thoughts and was really depressed. I was at rock bottom, as deep down as you could possibly be. I lost faith in everything. I tried to take my own life—twice.

Everything changed after the second attempt. I woke up at the local hospital, my neighbour found me. I don't know what happened, but something in my brain snapped. The only thing I wanted was to be **alive**. Maybe some sort of close death experience? I don't know. I stopped caring about anything negative in my life but damn, it was hard. Really fucking hard. I made really slow progress, but things went a little bit better. Still addicted to everything but my mindset went from "everything is pointless" to "I can't do this forever, something HAS to change." Time went by and by accident I found you guys.

25th August 2013—Rebirth!

It never came to my mind that porn, especially PMO could be something bad. I thought everyone would do it and everyone would be fine with it. I found this subreddit and read some success stories and was amazed at how much this little fapping thing could change you. This is my first and only shot at NoFap and I thought to myself that this fucking time, all or nothing, NoFap or death. I'm 21 years now and I want to restart my game called life. I needed to get rid of my addictions, my messy apartment, my shitty job, find some friends, find something to do in life, improve my appearance and maybe, someday find a girl who loves me as much as I love her. I said to myself that's a shit-ton of stuff to do, so I better get started not tomorrow, not next Monday, not next month. Not even in an hour. No "last cigarette", no "last drink". I started right there, right now.

I quit smoking, drinking alcohol, drugs and porn on the very same day I quit fapping. I sold every console and every game I had, sold my beloved PC and bought a Thinkpad x200 laptop—good enough for work, music and Internet but no graphics card so right now I can't even play games if I wanted to. I bought myself a gym membership, went to a skin doctor to get rid of my acne, read a lot about cooking and nutrition and quit all types of soda and fast food as well. I turned my life upside down.

As everyone of you knows, quitting an addiction is never easy. Not for you and not for me. These thoughts went through my mind every single day:
• This is pointless, why am I even trying?
• My old life wasn't THAT bad...
• A lot of people do drugs/smoke/drink. This can't be the reason why I am unhappy.
• Nobody will notice any changes, so why do I even bother?
• My efforts will fail just like everything failed in the past.

• Just one last fap/drink/shot/snort/hit can't be that bad, I mean only one in 2/3/4/5 weeks is a moderate consumption! Right?

I'm sure some of you have the same thoughts right now. Just don't, believe me. It is NOT worth it! I managed to fight my way to 100 days, one day at a time. It went easier and my confidence grew. Every aspect of my life improved. I was finally feeling normal. Not really happy, but at least not as depressed as before. The higher my day counter climbed, the more faith I had in myself. And here I am, triple digits!

December 2013—My life right now

Everything is good. I don't regret any of the decisions I made. My appearance improved and I even made some friends! 145 lbs now, aiming for that magical 150. I'm more confident than ever. NOTHING can turn me down right now, my mind is as sharp as never before. You know what they say? Damaged people are dangerous. They know they can survive. That is 100% true for me. I fought death and won (or at least didn't lose I would say). What in the world could stop me? What could life throw at me to hit me off guard? Everyday fears—what? A rejection? Stress at your job? Self-doubts? Pff! I laugh at those 'problems'! I wasted so much time already. Today I live my life to the fullest without letting fear stop me.

Right now I'm fulfilling my dream. I somehow was able to turn all my savings from $500 to $6k in just 3 months, and I quit my job, my apartment, sold ALL my stuff. I will fly to the other end of the world and try my luck there. On the second of February next year, I will fly to Australia—and never come back. Nothing but some money and a huge backpack with all my stuff. This will be the adventure of my life, some Alexander Supertramp shit if you want to. Let's see what life has to offer!

Despite my more-than-worse circumstances, I managed to change my life. If I could, so can you. Don't start tomorrow, start NOW. If there is something to do, do it NOW. It starts with doing dishes, laundry, that one project that doesn't need to be done til tomorrow or even next week. You will feel so much better after you've done it. You have to do all this stuff at some point, so why not right now?

This report is longer than I expected, but if just one of you reads it and gets the motivation to start moving, it was worth it. Thank you for reading. If you have any questions, feel free to ask me ANYTHING. I will help you as much as I can, I promise.

Kind regards,

K.V.

Anonymous:

At first I didn't want to tell my wife. Wanted to do this on my own. Not to mention I'm a man, and as part of this team as you likely know we aren't much for sharing our weaknesses. But after my first set back due to this miserable cold that is still weighing me down, I reset the clock, she walked in the room and I just started talking.

She asked if I thought I was addicted. For the first time ever I said, "Yes." Then it just all came flooding out. Not a whole lot of detail of where I had been, but what I believed had happened to me and why I needed to stop.

She thanked me for telling her. I told her I would need her help. The weight of the world has been lifted. I thought I could do it before, but now I'll have help, and if was from someone I was scared to involve.

"My marriage is now immeasurably happier"

Anonymous: So I've just completed my second 90 days. I started in May, but originally I was allowing edging. Having noticed a lot of guys not allowing this I decided to reset at 90 and go again without edging. And I have to say I found it easier. Any of you guys who are struggling to control the urges take note. If you're not allowed to touch your knob except to wash it or have a slash then you can't get carried away and relapse. Besides it's a bit like torturing yourself anyway.

Originally I started after very nearly getting caught in the act of PMO by my wife. It was, however, undeniable as to what I had been doing. My wife takes a very dim view of the sex industry (and rightly so) and is something of a feminist. She doesn't stomp around in Doc Martens and dungarees bemoaning the rights of oppressed women everywhere, she just believes that society has an unfavourable slant on women and how they are perceived. And I can't argue with her on that score.

So obviously there was much wailing and gnashing of teeth and some serious soul searching on my part. I have always loved my wife and felt dreadful that I had hurt her so much. I also now have a three-year-old daughter whom I adore, and I want her to look up to me. And obviously if you have a daughter you have to ask yourself the question, "If debasing herself for the gratification of men is not acceptable for my daughter, then why should it be for anyone else's?"

I also went to see a therapist for a few weeks to see if I could

123

untangle some knots. He was understanding and a great help.

Although I originally started this as a way to give up porn and get my relationship with my wife back on course, I actually ended up finding the NoFap thing very helpful. If you're not getting seedy kicks on the sly checking out Internet porn then you find your interest in real, healthy sex increases considerably. Much to the delight of both me and my wife. I think we've gone from once or twice a month to two or three times a week.

I still have urges, but they don't really bother me now because I made the decision to not masturbate, so I just try to put them out of my mind and get on with my day.

This forum has been a Godsend. When I first posted the response was fantastic and gave me a lot of strength to pull myself together. And as I've continued on my NoFap journey I've often found myself on here looking for advice and tips to help me. And when I thought I could I've offered my own advice.

I've also found running and physical exercise very useful. If I've been at home, horny, and with no lovely wife to aid me in my hour of need. I've thrown my running gear on and pounded up and down the canal towpath for an hour. I'm too knackered to be horny when I get back.

My only other tip is pretty self explanatory. The buck stops with you. If you don't exercise a modicum of willpower you will relapse. And then you'll feel S@&T and you'll have to start all over again.

My marriage is now immeasurably happier and I think my wife is beginning to find her trust in me again. My daughter is still the same, small and very entertaining.

So there it is. Not much in the way of sage advice. Just a condensed version of my little marital crisis and how I put it back on track again. With no small thanks to all you guys out there who helped me with your advice and encouragement. You are all total f*****ng stars! I shall continue to avoid playing with my johnson and I'll keep checking in. Stay strong fellow fapstronauts! And thank you all so much!! :D

My Father: A True Fapstronaut

Mike: I am 19 years old. Today is my first day of being a fapstronaut. My father is my inspiration. Since I can remember, my mother has had serious health problems resulting in at least one major surgery a year. To pay off these medical bills as well as my sister's and my own tuition, my dad works a great deal of overtime on the night shift at his job. He would work all night then sleep during the day.

On his few days off, he would understandably be too tired to do anything but watch TV and have a couple beers. He was always the stoic type. My sister and I wished we had more time with him and my mother, stuck inside almost always because of her health, grew increasingly lonely. Yet we understood because of all the sacrifices he made.

Then, 3 years ago, my mother discovered my dad had a PMO addiction. It soon came to light that he had since his teenage years. This was the final straw for her. Now, they fought almost daily and came to the brink of divorce. That same year he took a pay cut and my, now 5'6" 275lb, father caught a major blood clot that could likely have been fatal. It was then he decided to change his life and break his 30+ year addiction.

It's been two years since he made the change. My mother is still very ill, college is still expensive, and he still works odd, long hours. But he is not the same man. Today he is 53 years old. He is 100lbs lighter and all muscle. When he gets off his 10hr night shift at 7AM, he immediately does a 2hr workout. In his spare time he has rediscovered his love of gardening and created a beautiful garden around our home. Now he never drinks or has any PMO. He is now more open and I feel emotionally closer to him than I ever have before. Now he and my mother are rekindling their relationship and truly falling back in love.

Life is still hard, but my dad has rediscovered his passion for life and, more importantly, his love of himself. He isn't a superhero. He is a man. A man I'm damn proud to call my father. Today is day one. Time to follow his footsteps and become the man I want to be. If he can do it, so can I. So can YOU. Let's do it fapstronauts!

Anonymous:

I am INSANELY PROUD of my husband and all of you for doing this!!

It's been an amazing journey (almost 50 days!) filled with revelations, brutal honesty, tears, pain, joy and relief. We're stronger than we ever were now that there are only two of us in our bed!

I just wanted to say, ROCK ON Fapstronauts! You are a cut above the crowd. You're on another level of manhood! You're the future of masculinity and I really hope that the philosophy of NoFap spreads to all corners of the world so relationships can be healed, men can be men again and women can bask in the attention, love and unpolluted sexual desire of their husbands/boyfriends.

(oops! Don't want to forget the femstronauts! Rock on girls!!)

Losing my faith in God helped me overcome my porn addiction

BerlinSpecimen: Yes, this is a long post, but you know what, I feel like I earned it.

I've been waiting to do this for 90 days—no, much, much longer. I haven't gone 90 days in…honestly…I don't know if I've ever gone 90 days since the day when I first discovered fapping as a kid. If that sounds sad, it's because it is. Terribly, horribly sad. I didn't go 90 days when I was baptized at age 13, or when I spent all summer working as a camp counselor at a Christian summer camp, or when my grandpa died, or, just ever.

I've done a lot of bad things, but nothing has haunted me or made me feel worse about myself than fapping did. I used to hate myself. I had no hope of ever stopping, and that hopelessness bled into other areas of my life: physical health, relationships with people and with God, even just ever being happy.

So how did I ever overcome the one thing I never thought I'd solve? Let me tell you:

• I realized that I hate PMO. Really, deeply hated it.
• I accepted that I could like myself, if I could live with integrity.
• Most importantly, I lost my faith in God.

I don't want to discourage any religious readers here, but this is my true experience, and I'm proud of it. Losing my faith in God was painful and terrible and it was an incredibly depressing, but on the other side of that transformation, I no longer see my addiction as the influence of demons or the natural expression of my wicked sinful heart, but as a very human, very natural (albeit misplaced) desire for sexual intimacy. It was a bad habit reinforced by neurochemicals but nothing mysterious or ethereal. I lost faith in God and gained faith in myself. I didn't pray for power over sin; I realized that I already had the power to control my actions. And so I did. I realized that the life I wanted to lead was incompatible with PMO, so I simply made that decision. "Simply" doesn't mean easy, of course. Lust can dig into your chest and crush you in waves. But not resorting to PMO is not

126

complicated: just don't do it. So that's what I did.

I failed plenty of times, even after my "deconversion", until, finally, I didn't. It's easy for a few days, but terribly hard after a few weeks. For a while, my chest ached, I felt like throwing up, and I couldn't sleep. Triggers are unfathomably potent, and I had to take great care to avoid them. But once I got over that hump, it got easier again. I don't have those feelings anymore. I can see things on the computer or feel certain ways that would normally trigger me into a night of PMO, but now I can just move on. It's just wonderful.

Success in this area has given me the confidence to tackle other challenges. Since I've started this 90-day streak, I've lost over 20 pounds, I've started swing dancing, I joined a band, and I'm seeing a girl (don't call her a girlfriend, don't jinx it). I'm not talking about superpowers here, I'm saying that all this potential was already inside of me, trapped behind my addiction. No, girls don't wash over me like the breath of Zeus, but no longer do I talk to girls with the nagging shame of knowing that I jacked off to a porn star the night before, and in that sense, sure, I have more confidence.

I love myself. I look in the mirror, and I don't feel regret. I think this is how normal people feel. I hate the amount of time I've wasted feeling guilty and ashamed, but I get to look forward now with a clear conscience. I love my life.

And thank you all for indulging me in my 90-day victory rant!

Anonymous:

Around week 8 something magical happened: I was reading a book, when suddenly I noticed I was really aware. Not caffeine-aware, but little-kid-aware, if that makes sense. Like the only thing my brain cared about while reading the book was the book. Not the shit going on tomorrow, not the shit that happened earlier in the day, not worrying about getting laid off and not finding work, not worried about death or never owning my own house, not worrying if I worry too much, not worrying about blood pressure or eating carbs, and on and on. Remember when you were a little kid and could look at a leaf and just be completely amazed? The kind of amazement that geniuses never lose? I felt like I took two giant steps towards being in that state of mind again.

"For the first time since I was a child, I'm genuinely happy" (female)

infinitesimal: I thought when I reached 90 days of NoFap, I would have seen all the benefits of my experiment. At the six-month mark, life is only getting better.

To be fair, early on I started a meditation practice to teach my brain to control the urges. Every day now, I sit for at least ten minutes. It's a combination of meditating and NoFap that brought about all the great changes in my life.

Before I was always filling voids in my life. Masturbation was probably my biggest addiction, but shopping, food, alcohol, sex, TV and online dating all helped me stay in denial. When I slowly starting getting rid of my addictions, I was left with such horrible emotional pain. Meditating was a huge challenge. It forced me to unequivocally accept my reality, warts and all.

I've come to realize that you've got to get comfortable with the gaps in life. The silence between thoughts, the pause between breaths, the space between things. It's where the magic happens. Now, without that stillness, life feels bleak and hollow. I crave the downtime.

On the outside, I am so much more confident. I stand up for myself at work. I'm no longer a pushover. I don't take things personally the way I used to. I've really accepted that everyone has their own journey, not everything is about me.

Everything about sex is better. Orgasms come so much easier. I definitely get more attention from the opposite sex. I'm not as nervous when good-looking men talk to me. I'm getting better at making eye contact, flirting, and smiling.

Most importantly, I have empathy. I'm not afraid to connect with people, and I'm no longer pushing them away. All the relationships in my life are improving. I understand where others are coming from. It makes conflict resolution a breeze. Because I can grasp others' perspectives, I'm also not manipulated the way I used to be. There is so much less drama in my life. I've gone out and made some excellent friends. They feel like family and that's so important when you're single in a big city. Because I'm not lonely, I'm not binge eating. I've lost weight. I'm the best I've looked in years.

For the first time since I was a child, I'm genuinely happy. For me, NoFap was an amazing tool to start making things in my life right. The best way to describe it is it made me more human. Masturbating too often seems to reinforce the mentality of independence almost to a level of sickness. From what I can tell, my NoFap experiment has been a huge success. Much love fapstronauts!!!

How to make NoFap really, really easy (100 day report)

brick_eater: My last 100 days have been truly transformative. Since I first discovered NoFap back in the summer of 2012, I've been through both periods of strict abstinence and periods of indulgent binging, and it's taken me nearly two years to discover what the real secret to success with this is. My second-longest streak started on January 5th 2013 and lasted 90 days. Literally seconds after the 90th day passed, I took my eyes off the clock and loaded up my laptop. I'd been waiting for weeks to fap, and of course immediately after I did I felt fucking terrible. Despite feeling like shit I fell back into my old ways and readopted my self-destructive habits for a long while.

This is not how success with NoFap works.

Currently I'm on the 100th day of what has been by far the most life-changing and yet easiest streak yet. It's a streak that as of today has only lasted 10 days more than the 90-day streak last year, and yet this one has had a far more profound impact on my life. Why? Because I have conducted my life in the certainty that this streak has no end. 100 days ago, I masturbated for the final time in my life. There is a 0% chance that I will ever fap again.

What you have to understand is that NoFap is not something you do for a short period of time. If you say to yourself "I'm going to do the 90 day challenge" then what you're really telling your brain is that you're going to abstain for a period and then you'll get to "reward" yourself with binging after (crazy thinking, but we've all done this). You may instead tell yourself that you'll abstain for 90 days, you'll fap once as a reward, then you'll abstain for maybe 100 days more, fap once, abstain for 150 days, etc. But you and I both know that this **just doesn't happen.**

Written below is what you have to do to make NoFap really, really easy, and have incredible success with it. I implore you to do this **today**—right now if possible, though if you're reading this at work or at school then it would be best to wait until you have some free time alone, as this initially requires some serious focus and mental energy expenditure.

Are you ready? Here's what you must do:

YOU MUST MAKE THE *TRUE* DECISION TO NEVER, EVER FAP AGAIN.

The power of a true decision is a remarkable thing that I first read about in *Awaken the Giant Within* by Anthony Robbins. It is not what we normally mean when we talk about decisions. For example, you may make the 'decision' to give up smoking, but after a couple of weeks end up giving in to your nicotine cravings. What you have to understand is that what you had thought had been a decision was not a true decision—*you never made the decision to quit smoking in the first place.*

A true decision is some supernatural, Doctor-Who-esque shit, in that it has the power to *transcend time.* This might sound ridiculous but bear with me. When I made the true decision that I would never fap again, it was an incredibly liberating feeling, because *in that precise instant* I made all of the (relevant) possible future decisions all at once. For the rest of my life, I will never again have to decide whether or not to fap, because I already decided that fapping is an *impossibility*!

In a way, it's fucking terrifying. It's like you've been living your entire life aboard an aeroplane that's been circling above a beautiful landscape. You've had momentary glimpses of the land below but have always turned your head away in fear, convincing yourself that it's just an illusion. Only now do you notice the skydiving kit at the back of the aircraft, and a small thought begins to form in your brain: "what if...?"

Making a true decision is like jumping out of the aeroplane—scary as hell and there's no going back. If you break a NoFap streak, you haven't left the plane. Once you finally make that decision to improve for good, life becomes an exhilarating free fall. It takes raw psychological strength to do it, and you will encounter a lot of resistance at first, but if you can break through that self-imposed mental block, you will experience a freedom and optimism like never before!

Now, when I say that this will make NoFap really easy, I do not mean that you will never experience urges. Even as I type this my balls are aching pretty bad. So long as my dick continues to work, I don't think the urges will ever go away. But although you experience the discomfort of the urges, it is a discomfort that you just accept with grace and ease. Every time an urge arises, you look it square in the eye and, with UNFALTERING CONVICTION, you mentally declare the following word: **"No."** You have already made the decision that you will never give in; in that moment you are simply passing the message on from your higher consciousness to your lower consciousness. From

130

there you simply channel that sexual energy into whatever you were doing, and you do it with a new-found, controlled vigour.

You need to have a concentrated and brutally honest think about your life. Do you want to settle for mediocrity? If you're reading this then the chances are you don't. At a deep level, no matter how you rationalise it, you know that fapping is holding you back, and that *you must cut it out forever.* The time has come for you to decide whether you are going to condemn yourself to a life of indiscipline and self-indulgence or free yourself from the shackles of addiction and transform into something far greater than you had imagined possible.

Make the right decision. Make it a *true* decision. Make it today.

Jump off that fucking plane.

Anonymous:

One thing I had realized was that my flatline (at least toward the end) wasn't a flatline at all. It was change in thinking in regards to sexual excitement and arousal. Rather than relying on porn and mental fantasies to get my motor running, the only thing that gets me there now is the touch and feel of a real woman.

"Flashback"

Apeman: Here's who I was in college.

I enter the main hall. I carefully avoid the impulse to look at the ground; this is a sign of weakness. But I can't look anyone in the eye. It weirds me out. I feel like if we hold eye contact too long, I will come off as a creep. Of course I'm a creep. Odds are, I've just spent hours jerking it to weird, kinky pornography.

I get my food—healthy: fruits and vegetables and some lean protein. I stare at my food or scan the middle distance as the cashier rings me up. If the cashier says anything to me, I mumble some sort of reply and pray it's an appropriate response to whatever they said. God forbid I get tripped up saying "you too" to "enjoy that apple." Not again. I'll die.

I find a seat at an empty table. If I'm lucky, I'll spot a friend and can distract myself with their conversation as we eat.

But usually I sit alone, and there's nothing to distract me from scanning the room. I instantly pick out the hottest girls. I eat my lunch sullenly as I tell myself all the reasons I should go talk to one, knowing that I never will. I beat myself up for being a coward until I flee the building, retreating to my room to fall once more into the infinite porn abyss...

End flashback

What I kept realizing today was that I'm nothing like that guy. **Somewhere, seemingly without my realizing it, I became an entirely different kind of dude.**

I don't look away reflexively when I meet a stranger's eyes from across a room. I give them a friendly nod and a smile. Maybe a "how's it going?" if they're close enough.

I don't mumble something and stare into the distance when someone talks to me, ending the conversation and hoping like hell that one of us is able to leave. I look them in the eye and speak clearly. If neither of us are going anywhere, I try to get their story. Everybody likes telling their story, and I like to listen. You'd be amazed the kind of characters you cross paths with every day. Part-time smugglers and saints and serial killers and special forces agents and everything in between, all brushing shoulders as they navigate this strange world...Endless stories. I'm in love with this world.

And I don't spend upwards of 5 hours a day locked up by myself, surfing the net (and telling myself the feeble lie that I'm trying to learn something useful), playing videogames, and masturbating myself to sleep.

I'm meditating. I'm doing yoga. I'm learning to code a little (it's hard! But not as hard as I thought...) I'm paying off my loans by working down at the bar, and getting to know the stories of the regulars and my co-workers. Everyone is endlessly interesting if you pay close enough attention. I'm working out a ton.

And above it all, my heart overflows with gratitude for the myriad blessings of my life. There are things I wish were different sure, but even that is worth being grateful for! It keeps me striving and reaching. It keeps me moving. It keeps me alive. And if you've read this far, I'm grateful for you, too. More than you know.

I am still a far cry from my vowed goal of 150 days clean, but in this moment, I am Fapstronaut. And it is more than enough. For it has transformed my life. And I am intensely grateful for what this fight has given me.

90 day report—hardmode—from a female

Sammie83: I was addicted to sex, pornography, and masturbation. My fiancé has also been doing the NoFap hardmode challenge with me, as he was addicted also, but his 90 days was about two weeks ago. Here's how I've changed.

• I have friends.

• I can easily hold a conversation.

• Self-confidence has increased.

• My relationship with my fiancé is way beyond better than it ever was.

• I now have a relationship with my siblings.

• I find everyday things more enjoyable.

• I have nothing to hide on my electronics, so a large source of paranoia is gone.

• I'm completely happy.

These changes are in no way because I stopped watching porn. All these changes, including the hardmode challenge, grew from a desire to better myself. NoFap was not the catalyst, a desire to change was. I have no superpowers from not touching myself, I have superpowers from incredibly difficult, and diligent, work to get out of the rut of depression and addiction. I think many of us forget that it isn't stopping your addiction that gets you "superpowers", but your own will to change.

Will we continue hardmode? Until we get married next March, yes. We have made the decision that it is best if we wait.

Will we continue not watching porn? Certainly.

Will we continue NoFap? Until we're married, definitely. After then? We're not too sure.

Is it still as hard today as the first week/month? No. Eventually, I'd say around 2/2.5 months, my libido leveled out. I no longer crave porn/masturbation. I obviously still get aroused, but there's very little desire to take that arousal anywhere.

If you have any questions, especially gender-specific, feel free to ask! I'd love to help any men understand my journey or give advice to any ladies out there.

ElJefe's Journal (excerpts)

Jeff: October 31, 2013

I feel so depressed. Fucking flat. No libido, but that is the least of my concerns. No urges to fap, I HATE porn and I hate masturbation.

This is what I was covering up for so long by wanking, this feeling of emptiness and hopelessness. I feel void of all emotion. Today I was surrounded by people who didn't know about my depression or that there was even anything wrong with me. I had a singing lesson with a new teacher who doesn't know. I had to pretend but I was only just holding it together. The way everyone was felt overwhelming and I felt like I just wanted to get out of there, go somewhere with no people, and scream my absolute head off. I still want to scream. I also want to die. I know this isn't rational, though, because I'm getting better, and I've seen big improvements. But it doesn't change the fact that right now, in this very moment, I hate myself and don't feel I deserve to live. I'm just a lazy piece of shit cunt that can't even get his assignments in on time or get his dick up. I'm practically sub-human. URGH WHY AM I HURTING SO MUCH?! HOW IS THIS FAIR?!

Gonna go for a nap, or listen to some music about death, not that that'll help cessate it, it will just make me feel worse because I can't even cry right now.

January 2, 2014
Dear PMO,

You broke down my resolve and turned me into a crazed animal. You controlled me for six years and to say I have had enough of you would be an understatement. I am good, I look after my body, I eat healthily and I don't drink much or take drugs, but the one time I do on New Year's Eve, you come back to me the next day and the day after, begging with me, pleading with me to "just this once". Well, guess what, motherfucker, no. No you will not get anything from me "just this once" or ever. I will not "just have a wank, it's not as bad". I will not. How *dare* you try to tell me what to do like this?! Who do you think you are?! What authority do you have over me?! You do know don't you that every time you try to trick me like this I just get stronger. I transmute this energy you have given me and write a song, a poem, a letter, I practice singing or I meditate. Who's the bitch now, bitch? Not me, that's for sure. I'm going to reclaim my manhood and make love to beautiful women just like I should. I am a beautiful person, not a filthy lonely pathetic addiction like you are. You are not me, you tell me you are me but you are not. I am totally separate from you. You shocked me just now because you disappeared for a while and then you came back stronger. You think you are so clever. But you will not win, so you may as well give up. I know you won't give up just yet, but it's only a matter of time. I have won this war already. There will come a time very soon when you will just have to admit defeat. I'm all for peace but sometimes a man has to do what a man has to do for the sake of others. I'm not just doing this for myself, I'm becoming a better person so I can help others. I want you to know that I hate you more than I hate anything in this entire world, this is me crushing you. The more you try to crush me the more I will fight back. The more you try to beat me the more I will beat you. Fuck you, you despicable cunt. You cancer of the mind, evil to your very core. Fuck you.

Go suck a dick,

Jeff

January 2, 2014

That was probably the biggest urge I have ever had in my life. It was just so incredibly intense. I was honestly not in a place to have any rational thought, but somehow I noticed the tiny part of my rational mind that told me to take two minutes out to cool down, so I closed my laptop and sat down and meditated in front of my little Buddha shrine in my room. I only managed about five minutes because I was in such a dopamine frenzy, but it was enough to make me calm enough to stop me relapsing. I then went downstairs and started writing a song, and then I wrote that letter to PMO. It was a *very* close shave.

Obviously it was New Year's so we all got a bit drunk and maybe high. But that is one night of the year. If we're really serious about quitting PMO, we need to start drinking always in moderation, or if we think that impossible, we need to go teetotal. Probably better to avoid all other drugs completely. Don't fool yourself if you know you have no control over yourself when you have a hangover. You're doing this for yourself and for your future, not for a night out on the town when you get pissed, forget what you did, and relapse the next day. As Apeman would say, "do it for her, the mother of your children".

Next time you feel a relapse coming on, or you find yourself heavily triggered, try and find somewhere deep down that tiny voice that says "take a couple of minutes out" and do that. Sit down and just be aware of your mind and the state it's in. It'll be frantic and impossible to comprehend. It will be trying to make you touch your cock. Just watch it and be with it. Don't force anything. It absolutely worked for me. I'm not going to let this beat me. *Even* if I relapse, I will just get straight back up again without having batted an eyelid.

January 5, 2014

I will continue to maintain the right headspace and break out of this. Porn is what stole my manhood and I am now reclaiming it.

Never in my life have I felt this good and this in control of my life, and there is no way I am going to throw that away for momentary pleasures that are meaningless and lead to nothing but pain and despair. The more I don't fap, the more intelligent, interesting, witty and charming I feel myself become.

"HOCD rocked me to my core"

Kenny: Who I am: A 28-year-old regular guy. Started PMO when I was about 18. Feel free to read my story. I realize that this is a long post and I'm mostly posting this for personal reasons, to finally get it off my chest. Maybe someone out there can relate.

Before: On average I fapped about once a day. I didn't think this was excessive by any means—in fact I thought it was normal. I wasn't into weird fetishes or anything, but the porn had gradually become more intense and aggressive over the years. Unable to recognize it, I had developed several reoccurring anxieties. First and foremost when I was about 20 years old I started to have HOCD (homosexual obsessive compulsive disorder). This was extremely weird for me because I had been into girls my entire life. I can remember chasing and getting my first kiss from girls when I was about five or six years old. The HOCD rocked me to my core, and I developed anxiety over it fairly quickly.

A couple years passed and I was still PMO'ing every day. At this point I was 23 years old, and I met and became serious with a beautiful girl that I had met at the gym. After about a year of dating we got engaged to be married. We were crazy about each other and in love. Although things seemed to be going great we had some issues that quickly developed. I wasn't giving her enough attention. I constantly fantasized about other women. I was bartending at the time and had girls throwing themselves at me every day. I found myself wanting to PMO rather than have sex with my beautiful fiancée. Eventually it got to the point where she was so unhappy that she broke up with me, gave me back the ring, and moved out. I was beyond crushed. I cannot put into words what I went through mentally after this. I fell into a PMO marathon of sorts. Depressed, anxious, and although I fantasized about women CONSTANTLY the HOCD began to get worse and worse. At this point I had no idea what the porn was doing to my brain. I was unable to connect the dots with porn and the HOCD. I had never felt so alone in my entire life. I knew I wasn't gay but I couldn't get the compulsive obsession out of my head. Along with this

136

I developed a severe depression that I hid from everyone because I was so embarrassed about the HOCD. Suicide crossed my mind on a regular basis. I thought I was the only guy in the world going through this.

On the bright side, although I was going through mental torture I was still able to pursue my career and I landed a great job. However, the PMO and the anxiety was still there every day. The anxiety was starting to get worse and wasn't just related to HOCD. I had become anxious with many different aspects of my life. A couple more years pass by. I'm still single and still fantasizing and chasing girls around, dipping my toes into the pickup community. I become obsessed with chatting up and meeting new girls. My friends and family notice a huge change in me and my personality. All the while the HOCD is almost at a mind-crippling point. This was a weird dynamic that is really hard to explain. I wanted and fantasized about girls on a constant basis, but at the same time, the HOCD had me on the brink of suicide. I'm unable to form any attachment to the women I date. I changed the girls in my life faster than I changed my socks. I needed constant novelty. I broke a lot of hearts during this period in my life. As soon as I'd sleep with a girl I would want nothing to do with her. I hated this. All I wanted to do was to find the woman of my dreams. To make matters worse, my ex-fiancée had met and got engaged to be married to another guy. The only thing that remained constant in my life was the fact that I still PMO'ed every day. Nothing weird or crazy, just once a day. I began to become extremely needy with women as well. My entire self-worth was dependent on what the girls thought of me. I had turned into a PMO-fueled monster without realizing it.

Then one day I was browsing /r/askreddit, and a question that someone posted caught my attention. This guy asked "Why do I constantly objectify women?" I often asked myself the exact same question so I clicked on the link. I read a few negative responses, and then I noticed a guy posted a link to /r/NoFap and explained that he had been fap free for seven days. I went to the link and discovered this community. I read everything there was to read on "yourbrainonporn.com". At one point I started crying because I realized my prayers had been answered, and I realized what was at the root of my issues. Porn. And I had no idea. I immediately swore off porn and began my NoFap challenge.

After: 90 days later here I am. I can honestly say giving up porn was the best decision I've ever made. Shortly after starting my journey I met a girl, and things are going amazing. We're seeing each other exclusively now and I have no desire to move onto something else. I still fantasize some, but those thoughts are easily controlled now. And for the first time in years I can feel a healthy attachment being formed. We've only been dating for a couple months now, but I honestly feel like I may have met the woman I'm going to marry. The HOCD is almost completely gone, albeit a few spikes here and there. I'm no longer anxious or depressed. I cannot describe the difference in happiness. It feels like a 1000lbs has been lifted off my shoulders. I'm motivated and kicking ass in the gym and started eating healthy again. My boss has never been happier with my performance. Life seems bright and happy again, and I hope to continue my NoFap journey for the rest of my life.

Were all of my problems porn related? I don't know. All I know is how I feel now compared to 90 days ago. And it's a night-and-day difference. It wasn't easy. Early on the urges were intense, and I almost relapsed a number of times. It took a lot of willpower to stay clean. This community helped me the most and you guys always had my back. This is my story. If you have read this far, thank you. I mean that sincerely. Cheers.

I unintentionally got my boyfriend to stop looking at porn/fapping with wonderful results—please try...

Anonymous: I had been taking a lot of courses discussing some the psychological effects porn has on the brain (yay women's studies classes). I brought it up with my boyfriend as a topic of discussion ONLY because it was interesting—I wasn't trying to get my boyfriend to stop watching porn or jerking it, and at the time I was a porn viewer myself . However, unknown to me, my boyfriend quit porn/jerking as a result. He went from having major difficulties orgasming during sex (unless a BJ) to being able to orgasm multiple times in a single session. His sexual appreciation of me increased significantly as well—now it's as if every little thing I do turns him on, which is quite nice. Sex became much more personable as well. It wasn't until I commented on his sexual changes that he admitted to me that he felt that I may be right and that he had quit watching porn cold turkey after that conversation. He also said it was incredibly difficult but worth it.

I have had male friends before tell me about their difficulties enjoying sex but none have ever tried simply discontinuing porn/jerking because their refusal to admit it could be influencing sex at all. But as a girl who watched porn just as long as any guy, I'm telling you that it does have a huge impact on your sexual relationships. I stopped watching porn/having-me-time as well and I've noticed huge changes to my own sexual attitude: it used to be impossible to make me orgasm through clitoral stimulation unless I was the one doing it but now my bf can surprisingly easily. Sex has gone from feeling like someone is trying to jerk off into me to actually *having sex*.

Day 105: overcoming the greatest challenge of my life.

Anonymous: I have been through the valley of many of life's sickest and stickiest habits: alcohol, tobacco, marijuana, gambling and junk food. For some gambling and alcohol are mere recreation. For me they were consuming. My departure from the first three items listed was about twenty-five years ago. One habit, an addiction, has been with me since I was about eleven years old.

One hundred and five days ago I made a decision to turn away from porn and masturbation completely, for good. Thanks to the commitment and the help I've received from this forum I've upheld that commitment. For the first time in my life I am free of porn and masturbation.

The first thing I did when I came to this forum was to read about the benefits of life without PM. That's how I've overcome every bad habit I've ever had. I think about the consequences that I'm experiencing because of the bad habit, I focus my attention on the benefits I'll gain by leaving the bad habit behind, then I make the decision to go in the opposite direction and I keep going. Is it just that simple? Not always. Sometimes—in fact most of the time—there's a little voice that reminds me of the immediate pleasure or reward that the bad habit delivers. There was a period that preceded my change in which I was on and off with PM. The definite decision and this forum helped me through the transition.

Now that I've moved on I realize that one slip could wipe out everything I've accomplished. I've experienced this with every bad habit or addiction I've overcome, and I'm determined to not allow that to happen with this addiction or any of my past addictions. There is no such thing as just once. I'm fifty-five years old and for the first time in my life the blinders are off.

Not only am I free of this soul-stealing habit, I am as healthy as

I've ever been. I do yoga every day. I eat a plant-based diet. I'm living life on my own terms. Thank you to all who have helped me. For those who are feeling the worthlessness that this habit can cause, realize that you can make a firm decision and put this behind you if you simply focus on the benefits you'll gain by arresting the habit, focus on the consequences you bring by allowing it to continue, and stop! The pain of craving your habit happens in the moment. Realize that it's only a moment, and get out of the moment. Do something, don't stay in that moment. Your pain will dissolve, you'll find yourself doing something else, and the moment will have passed. Each time you move beyond the moment it gets easier, and the moments become less frequent until you get to the point where they all but dissolve.

When the pain of addiction dissolves you're left with clear vision. You realize that a picture is not a woman. You stop giving a damn about what people think. What do you think? That's what matters. You realize beautiful women are everywhere, and they're just people. I'm starting to babble so it's time to move on. So much has changed in a hundred and five days that I can't begin to describe how different things are. Take the plunge. You'll begin feeling better immediately and it keeps getting better and better. The pain I described passes so quickly you'll kick yourself for having carried the bad habit. But so what. The habit is gone and you are free. What could be better?

Anonymous:

The MOST IMPORTANT thing you can do for your recovery is to GIVE to others in recovery, and I've found no place better than here [NoFap]. YOUR opinion and experiences are valuable to others here, no matter how freaky or "unique". In fact, the more oddball your experience, the more likely you will help that other oddball that is just like you and feels totally alone. YOUR support matters to someone else here, no matter how small or weird you feel on any given day.

"Porn isn't always 'no big deal'"

sea_warrior: I am a lady who from my teenage years was always very sexually eager and curious. I watched a good amount of porn and was psyched to "finally" lose my virginity at 17. I dated guys, slept with guys, had a couple (dysfunctional) relationships but nothing long-term enough in my "adult" years to really explore sex in a committed relationship context. But I would never have imagined *ever* having a problem with a boyfriend watching porn. It was just something people did to satisfy momentary urges and explore their sexuality. No big at all. The idea of getting angry about it would have just seemed silly and pointless.

I entered my first long-term relationship at 23. Never did I think it would turn into that, because he was a little older—6 years and change—and we were coworkers, so it seemed more suitable for the fun sexy fling category. I didn't see him in that "boyfriend material" way. But we clicked emotionally and intellectually enough that things started to roll forward from there, first to a commitment to monogamy, then to official BF/GF status, which was exciting and new and weird for me. But he was a serial monogamist, so such things weren't as scary for him. :)

Pretty much everything was great at first, but then problems started to emerge with our sex life. First, I was in that fun "honeymoon" phase and was always pawing at him, wanting to fool around, or fuck, or whatever. He would as often as not brush me off, sometimes thinking I was just messing with him, or maybe he was tired, or maybe he was more interested in watching the movie/TV show that was on. Whatever it was, there was always a reason. So his response rate was not great, and he almost never initiated sex—maybe a couple times a month, and this while we were spending 3-4+ nights a week together. And we couldn't communicate about sex either—he couldn't talk openly about my needs, his needs, or how to bridge the gap between the two.

In addition to this, he had a really hard time expressing his attraction to me. For whatever reason. In the very beginning, there were a few little flattering comments here and there, but they faded away fast. Women on TV or in magazines or even other guys' girlfriends could be "hot"—but not me. I would put effort into a sexy outfit and instead of calling it what it was, he would make a wisecrack and deflect somehow. Or just look confused, like me dressing sexy and wanting to do it was a "change in plans" that had to be pondered over and digested before he could respond positively. This was baffling because past boyfriends had always complimented frequently and sincerely. I had *always* felt sexy up to that point, no matter if my clothes were on or off.

Add those two things together and the insecurities started to grow at an alarming rate. Of course, when I brought them up, his answers were "Insecurity is an unattractive quality" or "You shouldn't care if I find other women attractive, it's inevitable" or "Why would I even be with you if I didn't find you attractive?" None of this was untrue or illogical, strictly speaking, but it didn't address the core issue: that he wasn't communicating his attraction to me in words OR actions. That I felt "invisible" to him sexually, and that by wanting sex, more often than not I felt I was pestering him. That I didn't feel desired by the one person who was supposed to desire me most, to make me feel beautiful and sexy and adored.

Now throw this into the mix: one day I picked up his phone to set a picture of me as his wallpaper—just as a joke, nothing weird—and discovered a huge folder of porn clips featuring other women. Sorted by first name. I didn't snoop—they were right there when I picked it up. He had barely if ever mentioned porn before, so I hadn't had a chance to wrap my head around the idea—and now my physical and sexual insecurity was thrown into the stratosphere. He seemingly only tolerated sex with me, *never* made me feel sexy…and at the same time had collected all these clips of other women??? It was heart-breaking and confidence-shattering. Especially for me, a previously *extremely* confident person who had never thought there was anything wrong with her wanting sex in the least. It wasn't that he had a low sex drive, I realized—it was that he preferred porn to sex. He preferred images of these other women, these strangers with their clothes off, to me. Half of me was devastated and wanted to curl into a ball and cry forever— and half of me was furious. I mean *furious*. Drive-around-the-block-so-I-could-scream-inside-my-car-at-the-top-of-my-lungs furious.

After months of back-and-forth about sex, porn and insecurities, including some really vicious fights and intense cry-fests, I finally reached a place where I had to ask him to stop watching porn. We had to *try*, at least, to see if this was a way to reprogram our sex life as a couple, his ability to express attraction to me and my ability to feel secure and wanted. Believe me, I was asking myself all the time if he was capable of giving me what I needed at all or if it was a waste of my time. I wondered if it was fair to ask that of him. But I knew that ultimately if he wasn't willing to make the sacrifice, I shouldn't be willing to continue the relationship. In my heart, I knew my complaints were valid and he should want to improve the situation however possible, up to and including abstaining entirely from porn use. Without both his willingness and ability to change, the long-term life we were planning together was pointless. I simply couldn't go on in our relationship without a dramatic change.

So he stopped using porn. And guess what? He started initiating sex a *ton* more, groped me on the couch during movies instead of pushing me away, was more vocal and generous in bed than he had ever been before. He also started complimenting me *way* more, even calling me sexy—something he never had before. He told me what he wanted in bed, and made a bigger effort than ever before to give me what *I* wanted. Things didn't change overnight, but they changed dramatically in a matter of months, after years together. We still have a long way to go with our sex life, and I'm a long way from feeling confident enough to—gasp—watch porn together, though we have in the past, or see him openly ogle other women without getting upset, but enormous strides have been made. Due in such large part to him abstaining from porn.

Now, this is only my experience. I'm not saying that cutting porn out of your life is some magic bullet for fixing every relationship issue ever. But it sure as shit repaired a bunch of things about our relationship that were really dysfunctional. Deep-seated issues with pornography are rarely isolated to that topic—often they stem from other things, like a lack of communication surrounding sex and attraction in a relationship, for example. For me it was a complex cocktail that was as much about the secrecy, shame, and selfishness surrounding it as the actual fact of it. I don't doubt that two people in a relationship watching porn together could actually *improve* their sex life, or that porn could benefit them as individuals in various ways. None of that is wrong on any objective moral level. But porn isn't always "no big deal". Sometimes it really is a big deal. And sometimes it isn't wrong to make it go away for the sake of your relationship.

Tom:

I've always been the type of guy who would be uncomfortable in the real world. There have been many times when I would not leave the house for weeks at a time because it was easier to stay in my room where I couldn't potentially find myself in a bad situation, judged or laughed at. I have been that way for the majority of my life. I could and would go out only if truly necessary, but I would try and justify staying in and canceling or making pitiful excuses to my friends as to why I can't see them as planned.

I am only on day 8 of NoFap, and today I walked out of my house, got on a bus, went to a crowded mall for no reason whatsoever and

143

loved every damn second of it. There was no hesitation in doing all that; it just happened and I went with it. It usually took me hours, even days to mentally prepare for something like that. I blamed it on being an introvert, but now I'm not so sure. So far, every day of NoFap seems to provide yet another gift—Whether it's physiological or simply placebo, I don't care. I like this.

I held my head high, talked to people, smiled at strangers and walked tall in a sea of people in a busy shopping mall :)

Femstronaut at 35 days

Tatiana: First of all, sorry for not being super active in this community. I lurk a LOT, almost daily, and I'd like to say a massive THANK YOU to everyone for sharing your ups and downs. The thoughtful reflections and insights have kept me motivated.

So, I started NoFap after watching The Great Porn Experiment, and after browsing the NoFap reddit I figured, hey, this might work for me. I was unmotivated, frustrated and constantly going in and out of bouts of depression. I was PMOing every day and sometimes I would just lie in bed and do it for hours. I knew there was a lot that I wanted to accomplish but everything just felt stagnant. So I gave NoFap a go.

The first day was awesome. I went for an 11km bike ride, wrote a list of things to do and effortlessly ticked each one off. Cool things that have happened in the last 35 days:
• Offered two jobs based on personality alone.
• No more bullying at work.
• Raised $4000 for a not-for-profit.
• Took on more responsibility for the community organisation I am involved with, getting more respect.
• Confronted mother on unresolved family issues. She ended up flying my father across the country so that my family could be together for the first time in two years.
• Start training tomorrow for a half marathon in August; I have never done anything like this before!

What's interesting is that it doesn't take as much to turn me on now. I came across a photo of a guy in a suit the other day that normally wouldn't have had too much of an impact but I actually felt crazy from looking at it. I'm doing this on HardMode, and I'm hoping that NoFap will help me orgasm a lot easier when I'm with the next guy. This is usually a huge mission and probably because I was of the attitude that "It's just easier if I do it on my own."

Why does NoFap work? I honestly think that there is a lot to be said for discipline. Getting disciplined in one area makes it easier to get disciplined in other areas of life. Also, it's an escape from stress and pain that I can no longer use, so I have to do something else with all that energy. I did feel worse at stages, but it was weird, like I had a lot of clarity and could articulate and experience my pain more directly.

I have committed to the 90-day challenge, but I know it would probably be beneficial to keep going longer. Keep up the great work fapstronauts and femstronauts!!

"I'm loving life and you should too"

thomas123: After failing over and over again for as long as two years, I finally reached the 90 day milestone! My life has changed so much that I decided to reflect back on my teenage years to share how I was before porn, during and after. It will be a long read, but in my opinion my story should give hope. I will tell you how a popular happy, maybe chick-magnet kid turned into a fat foreveralone teenager in high school whose life completely collapsed because of porn. No attention from girls, extreme shyness and terrible grades were some of the things I had to deal with everyday. However I will first describe what kind of person I was before porn, because I believe that's the person you'll eventually turn into again after you're no longer addicted. If you're not interested in the first part, just read the 13-17 and 17-19 part to read about my struggle and when I discovered NoFap.

Age 0-12: Life was beautiful!

People described me as a funny, handsome, smart and athletic kid when I was growing up. I made a lot of friends in primary school and even some girlfriends. In the Netherlands (where I'm from) they start teaching you reading at age 6-7 usually, and they measure your progress in levels 1 to 10, 10 being the level when you mastered it. Anyway, my school was shocked to find out I reached level 10 in the first week of school when I was 6. I was even in the school newspaper, being the first kid in 10 years to accomplish this so fast. I started reading when I was 4 and could read big books for 14-year-olds when I was 5-6. They gave me extra homework and reading material, and I had to teach other kids to read as well. My other grades were also excellent, never scoring lower than A's on all tests. I was the top of my class, but I didn't really know what was going on because it all felt natural to me and easy. I was also selected for the top team of my local football (soccer) club when I was 11. It was a soccer club with 1400 members so it was quite an accomplishment. Everyone wanted to be my friend, and I even had girls standing outside my house after school every day because I was so popular and friendly. I was intelligent, popular, athletic and most of all I was happy. Life couldn't be any better. But then it was time to go to high school and my whole life changed.

Age 12-17: Life collapsed and I fell into the deep dark hole called porn addiction.

I already had seen some pornographic images when I was in primary school, but I didn't really know what it was and thought it was disgusting. However when I was 12, I started looking at more porn. I remember the rush I got was unbelievable; it's probably what heroin feels like. I did not know how to masturbate though, so I didn't get addicted to it at the time and wasn't watching very often. But it started to have some effects on me that I didn't see. I continued having great grades in my first year of high school, but there was something that was bothering me. I started to become more shy. I asked my parents about it, and they said it was a normal process of growing up.

Fast-forward to the summer when I turned 13. That was the day that marked the beginning of my terrible teenage years. I discovered how to masturbate and my first session I already was using hardcore porn. I still remember the scene crystal clear to this day. My first orgasm was the best feeling I had ever experienced. As you can imagine, I wanted that feeling over and over again. I started watching a bit more hardcore videos but not to the point of it being straight up extreme (yet). The effects of porn were becoming more clear at school, because my grades crashed. I had no motivation anymore and my concentration was beyond terrible. I started getting picked on because I was talking slow as well and because of my bad grades. This kick-started an addiction circle: the more I got depressed, the more I watched porn. My performance in my soccer games were also beyond pathetic. My stamina was gone and my confidence in the field too. I was already kicked out of the top team when I was 13. Furthermore I wasn't saying much to other players, and when I did, I spoke in a mumbly, stuttery way. I also got laughed at because of this. The coach put me in a position on the field that's basically useless. This was also the period when I got my first job at a supermarket. And you may have guessed it, I was VERY quiet there too and people took the piss out of me a lot there as well. I couldn't stand up for myself anymore. I started looking at more extreme videos that were very violent, all at age 14-15 before even having my first kiss. My friends were gone and the ones that sticked were making fun of me. I was sheltering myself in my room every day, because I was too scared to go outside. My family noticed something was different about me but they figured it was just a part of puberty. I also read on the Internet that masturbation and porn were healthy, so I didn't know what the hell was going on.

When I was 16 I started going to the gym to battle my confidence issues and social anxiety. I started getting bigger and people were commenting on my physique in a positive way. But then I decided to bulk and I took it way too far. I gained 40 lbs of fat in three months, and that year, when I was 16, was the darkest year of my life. I cried a lot before going to sleep, developed a video-games addiction and quit playing soccer. I had no friends. No attention from girls. I spent the whole year inside and I went to zero parties. I was on the brink of suicide and I had terrible depression. Thinking about it now, still gives me light shivers. I had hit rock-bottom, at least that's what I thought. My life got a bit better when I lost the 40 lbs again in three months, but I still had zero confidence, social anxiety, and no real friends. In August 2011 I discovered a thread on the misc section of bodybuilding.com, and that discovery changed my life.

Age 17-19: Climbing out of a dark hole.

I tried the NoFap challenge only as a challenge. I didn't expect to gain any results from it. I made it two days my first try, and that shows how addicted I was. I didn't try anymore after that moment, and three months later I discovered "yourbrainonporn.com". I started reading about the symptoms of porn addiction and my jaw dropped. I had ALL the symptoms that were described on this site:

• My friends were drifting away. I gave up hangouts to sit in my room and pleasure myself.

• My eyes looked dead and without color .

• Memory and concentration was terrible; it was almost as if I had dropped 30 IQ points.

• I had no girlfriend.

• I had an enormous amount of anxiety with human interactions in general.

• Muscle gains were slow as opposed to now.

• Literally NO energy. I slept 10-12 hours a night and I still had big black bags underneath my eyes. I always needed to sit down after standing for like 10 minutes, no exaggeration.

- I was terribly depressed and suicidal.
- I didn't feel "masculine".
- I felt the need to masturbate but it wasn't because of my libido.
- I could still masturbate without porn but it was very difficult.
- I was stressed, anxious, confused, had no goals in life.
- I couldn't defend or stand up for myself.
- I was basically "existing" but not living.

I was very euphoric that I finally found the source of my problems. I started following the advice on the site and tried to block porn out of my life. As I already expected, I made it in streaks of four to five days a time. But the people at school were starting to notice I was changing. Concentration and focus were coming back, and my grades were going up. A girl out of my class also was interested in me, but I still didn't know how to handle it. I did get my first kiss from her during school prom, and I was very happy. I made it three weeks without porn in January 2012, and I actually was scared how much effect abstaining had. I did have a very bad withdrawal. I had nightmares about porn, headaches, and I felt sick the times after I relapsed. But my life was slowly getting better. I went to Spain on vacation with my friends, and I felt like a huge chick magnet, making out with lots of girls while going out. That week in Spain was the best week of my life. I also graduated high school despite teachers saying I probably wouldn't make it. I started reading finance and investing books. I even sold my Playstation 3, because my video-game addiction was gone. I thought I was cured. But I was wrong.

The next year I took a year off from school, because I still wasn't sure what major to choose in university. I was sitting at home a lot and, as you can probably imagine, my addiction started coming back. I'll keep this part short. I started looking at more extreme porn than ever before and I almost committed suicide. From April to August, I started having three-to-four week clean streaks. Then in August of 2013, I relapsed for the last time until now.

Age 19-: I'm back and better than ever.

When I started university in September, I felt like a new person. I was making friends with total strangers, and my motivation was through the roof. I scored A's on all tests, and the school asked me to participate in their honours program. I also needed less sleep with my days scheduled from 6:45 till 23:45 sometimes, and I wasn't even tired. My muscle gains in the gym were through the roof, and I could eat a ton more than when I was younger and not gain fat. I had a pool party in September, and everyone was commenting on how much I had changed. I was so confident, and my voice was way deeper. Then on 21-11-2013 I finally reached 90 days PMO free! A quick summary of the benefits I experienced:

- Confidence is through the roof.
- Social anxiety is almost non-existent .
- Girls that I considered out of my league are now checking me out.
- I'm the person now that people come to if they have problems.
- I feel like a leader.
- I have a burning desire to achieve greatness, and I really mean burning. I aspire to be a legend like Napoleon, Newton and Caesar.
- My motivation is unbelievable.
- Random boners and morning wood are now a daily thing.
- Depression is gone.
- Random people start a conversation with me.
- I only need 8 hours of sleep to function.
- Sparkle in eyes and my face "glows".
- Concentration and memory are unbelievable—almost feels like I have a photographic memory.

I could go on forever, but these are the major benefits I've noticed. There were many times I wanted to give up on this journey; I've relapsed maybe 80-100 times. The process of quitting was VERY hard. There were moments I literally felt sick because the cravings were so bad. I just want you to realize that porn addiction is real and very dangerous and give you hope that it is 100% fixable. I hope that in 5 to 10 years mainstream medical science will recognize this problem and educate people about it. I also started a self-development website called "www.builttoachieve.com". It's still in the making, but my purpose with this site is to help people battle porn addiction, help bullied teens get their life back, and generally improve the quality of life for people. Because I'm loving life and you should too. Thanks for reading.

ThouShallNotPorn:

You have to make the commitment. No halfway shit. This is forever, there is no choice. There is no going back. Don't tell me you can't do it. There are many success stories. If you can't do it, then I think at some level you're not ready to quit porn. It's up to you to find out how to get there.

Additional resources

(For a complete and updated list, visit my website,
"AddictedToInternetPorn.com")

Books

-*The Willpower Instinct* by Kelly McGonagall. McGonagall, a psychology professor at Stanford, brings her classroom to the page in this exploration of desire and self-control. She draws a variety of willpower strategies and tactics from the latest in willpower science and explains how you can apply these techniques to any "I will," "I won't," or "I want" challenge in your life. A must-read for those of us whose greatest enemy is ourselves.

Your Brain on Porn: Internet Pornography and the Emerging Science of Addiction is Gary Wilson's recently released summary of porn addiction research, science, and experiential data—an excellent source for anyone interested in this topic.

-*Fortify*. This text is directed specifically toward adolescents and teens who are struggling with a porn addiction. Authored by Fight the New Drug, an organization committed to educating and arming today's youth against the dangers of Internet porn.

-*Love You, Hate the Porn: Healing a Relationship Damaged by Virtual Infidelity* by Mark Chamberlain and Geoff Steurer. This text addresses handling a pornography or cybersex addiction specifically within a committed relationship, including many inspiring stories of real couples and essential advice both for the addict and for the addict's partner. With this book, couples have the power to access a deeper level of trust and intimacy than they have ever shared, leaving no room for porn.

The Demise of Guys: Why Boys Are Struggling and What We Can Do About It by Philip Zimbardo and Nikita Duncan. Zimbardo, perhaps the nation's most famous psychologist, reveals the alarming downward trend of males in the modern world, demonstrating how over-medication, over-parenting, addiction to video games and pornography, and other factors are contributing to our downfall.

Dirty Girls Come Clean by Crystal Renaud. *Dirty* is one of the few texts to focus on female porn addicts, and it is very valuable for sharing many women's stories of addiction and recovery. Note that this book is written from a Christian perspective, which may turn away some readers.

Online Support Communities

"Your Brain Rebalanced" is a public forum for "Overcoming Pornography Addiction and Porn Induced Erectile Dysfunction", as well as all other problems related to compulsive porn use. This forum is an ever-growing and positive support community that includes general discussion as well as spaces for journals, success stories, female porn addicts, partners of porn addicts, etc.

"NoFap" is a movement that challenges people to "partake in the ultimate challenge" by abstaining from masturbation for a determined amount of time. NoFap began as a small group of men who wanted to increase their motivation by keeping their hands out of their pants, but it has since incorporated recovery from porn addiction and now boasts more than 100,000 members on its Reddit forum.

"Reuniting" is dedicated to exploring "the connections between sexual behavior, neurochemistry, and relationship harmony" and features a wealth of information and discussion about karezza, or *coitus reservatus.*

Websites, videos, and articles

"AddictedToInternetPorn.com" is my own website. It contains additional recovery advice, updates on my own journey, and reviews of recent research on porn addiction.

"YourBrainOnPorn.com" is the single most complete resource for up-to-date information on all aspects of Internet porn addiction and recovery.

"The Great Porn Experiment" is an informational talk on the rising wave of Internet porn addiction given by Gary Wilson, creator of "yourbrainonporn.com". An excellent place to start for an overview of the science of addiction and the personal and societal impacts of compulsive porn use.

The American Society of Addiction Medicine's "Public Policy Statement: Definition of Addiction" is a valuable read for anyone looking to understand the behaviors common to all addicts.

Dr. Eric J. Nestler is an expert on the neurological impacts of addiction, and he explains some of the common threads between substance and behavioral addictions in his article, "Is there a common molecular pathway for addiction?"

The Guardian published the article "Why more and more women are using pornography" in 2011, revealing that porn addiction is not just a man's vice.

Porn on the Brain is a British television segment on Internet porn's effects on today's youth, featuring the emerging research from Cambridge University that demonstrates physical changes in the brains of porn addicts.

Recovered porn addict Gabe Deem started the online community "Reboot Nation" to help others struggling with similar issues. His videos give a very helpful first-person account of porn addiction and recovery.

In November of 2005, Dr. Jill C. Manning gave testimony before a United States Senate subcommittee "On Pornography's Impact on Marriage & the Family". In this submission of evidence, Manning reviews and analyzes years of research studies, concluding that "Internet pornography is altering the social and sexual landscape. While there is much more to learn about these shifts regarding their impact on marriages and families, the research currently available indicates many negative trends."

In "Disclosure to Children: Hearing the Child's Experience", Black, Dillon, and Carnes explore the effects of a parent's sexual addiction on his or her children. A must-read for any porn-addicted parent or parental partner of a porn addict, especially one who needs guidance in communicating with children about the problem.

"How I fixed my porn-ravaged love life" is my own thread (under the name Spangler) on "yourbrainrebalanced.com" that contains my complete story. Read it or the other journals on the site if you are looking for detailed accounts of recovery.

Software

"Adblock Plus" is a free extension for the free web browser Firefox. With it, you will no longer have to worry about pop-ups or banner ads triggering and distracting you. It makes the Internet a whole lot nicer.

"K9 Web Protection" is a free software that blocks most explicit and dangerous websites, as well as keeping a log of every website visited. K9 is marketed as protection for children—which it does—but it is also useful for the recovering addict who wants to throw up as many roadblocks as possible against relapse. Though K9 is highly rated, know that no filter is perfect. And if you do not trust yourself with the power to deactivate K9, you can trust a friend with the password.

"Covenant Eyes" is marketed as an Internet accountability tool more so than a filter like K9, though it does provide that service as well. Covenant eyes requires you to log into the software in order to access the Internet, and then it periodically sends reports of your online activity to whomever you select as an accountability partner. This way you still have the choice of indulging your online whims, but you will have to explain them later, and your trusted partner can know when you need help getting back on the right track. Covenant Eyes costs $8.99-$12.99 per month.

Thanks for reading.

If you know of anyone who could benefit from this book, please send them to my website "AddictedToInternetPorn.com" for more information and continually updated news and resources. If you would like to contact me and get my help personally, you can also reach me at that website, where I respond to questions by email and video as my schedule allows.

You have my best, my friend.
Noah B.E. Church

84900272R00095

Made in the USA
Lexington, KY
26 March 2018